The Principles of Successful Awake Craniotomy

Ahmad Pour-Rashidi • Judith Aarabi
Editors

The Principles of Successful Awake Craniotomy

Perioperative Tips and Tricks

Springer

Editors
Ahmad Pour-Rashidi
Department of Neurosurgery
Sina Hospital
Tehran University of Medical Sciences
Tehran, Iran

Judith Aarabi
Community College of Baltimore County
School of Health Professions
Baltimore, MD, USA

ISBN 978-981-99-2984-9 ISBN 978-981-99-2985-6 (eBook)
https://doi.org/10.1007/978-981-99-2985-6

This Springer imprint is published by the registered company Springer Nature Singapore Pte Ltd.
The registered company address is: 152 Beach Road, #21-01/04 Gateway East, Singapore 189721, Singapore

Foreword

Brain surgery is challenging because of the complexity of the human central nervous system (CNS). Therefore, with the aim of preserving quality of life of patients, neurosurgeons should better understand the organization of the functional networks at the individual level before to excise a part of the CNS affected by a brain disease such as tumor or epilepsy. To this end, achieving cerebral mapping is of utmost importance in order to tailor the resection according to the cortical hubs and white matter tracts critical to maintain normal conation, cognition, and behavior. Even though noninvasive neuroimaging may provide interesting insights regarding cerebral processing, this technology suffers from major limitations. In fact, besides the lack of reliability, functional MRI is intrinsically not able to make the distinction between essential neural structures which must be surgically preserved from compensable regions which could be removed with the goal of optimizing the extent of resection. In the same spirit, tractography is incapable of giving direct functional information with respect to the axonal fibers—but represents only an indirect mirror of their anatomical distribution. As a consequence, awake surgery with intraoperative identification of the eloquent cortical-subcortical circuits by means of direct electrostimulation mapping combined with online neurocognition assessment throughout the resection remains the gold standard to maximize the benefit/risk ratio of brain surgery.

In this book, the authors detail the history, rationale, methodology, and results of CNS surgery in awake patients, by insisting on the need to build a multidisciplinary team with the goal of increasing the reproducibility of such a procedure under local anesthesia. Indeed, the pivotal role of constant interactions between neurosurgeons, neuroanesthesiologists, neuropsychologists, speech therapists, and neurophysiologists is emphasized. Integration of multiple talents around the patient is mandatory to explore the dynamics within and between brain networks in real time into the operative theater, and to adapt the surgical strategy based upon the comprehension of the individual functional connectome. Ideally, such a "connectome-based resection" should go beyond a classical surgical act, by being the ultimate product of strong relationships across fundamental neurosciences and clinical implications. Only an improved knowledge of CNS processes, especially by breaking with the traditional localizationist dogma to evolve towards a networking theory of neural functions, will allow an optimization of the outcomes following brain surgery.

Led by the editor, Ahmad Pour-Rashidi, this collection of work aims to serve as a comprehensive textbook for all physicians, offering a personalized approach to CNS surgery. I have no doubt that this comprehensive volume will be very helpful not only for neurosurgeons but also for all specialists involved in cerebral mapping in awake patients.

Hugues Duffau

Department of Neurosurgery
Gui de Chauliac Hospital
Montpellier University Medical Center
Montpellier, France

Institute of Functional Genomics of Montpellier
INSERM U1191
Montpellier, France

Contents

History of Awake Craniotomy <Awake Craniotomy, History>

Hadi Digaleh and Mahshid Fallahpour

1 Introduction

Simple skull trephination is one of the oldest invasive procedures dating back as far as 12,000 years for therapeutic intentions [1]. Currently, this intervention still exists in the Kisii tribe of Kenya, the *Omobari omotwe* (head surgeon), undertakes craniotomy on an awake patient for posttraumatic headache with dedicated specialized surgical tools [2]. Many trephined skulls that belong to pre-Colombian South America, Neolithic Europe, ancient Persia and prehistoric Africa were found and described since Broca's first impression [3]. Questions have been raised about trephination tools, indication and procedures in these remote regions over time. Since literature concerning the prehistoric era is lacking and existing evidence is inadequate, a comprehensive review is not feasible.

The original version of the chapter has been revised. A correction to this chapter can be found at https://doi.org/10.1007/978-981-99-2985-6_11

H. Digaleh (✉)
Department of Neurosurgery, Tehran University of Medical Sciences, Tehran, Iran

M. Fallahpour
Department of Public Health, San Diego State University (SDSU)-University of California San Diego (UCSD), San Diego, CA, USA
e-mail: mfallahpour3792@sdsu.edu

2 Awake Trephination in the Ancient Era

Trephination remains have been discovered all around the world and the amalgamation of these diverse practices can be marked in some regions. Specifically, T-shaped frontal burrs are common in Neolithic Europe which are trephined skulls that have influenced Arabic trephination in North Africa and the Canary Islands; however, it differs from the evidence found in East Africa. The shape of cranial openings is a surgical fingerprint and distinguishes regional origin. As such, arc-shaped and halo-shaped burr-holes, considered to be therapeutic interventions, have been found in China [4]. Moreover, pre-Colombian Peruvian cranial bones were analyzed indicating rectangular, cylindrical-conical and circular craniotomies [5] (Fig. 1).

Interestingly, there was also a great variation in the indications and purposes of trephination. The most practical and evidenced intention was therapeutic intervention of individuals who sustained traumatic assault and/or evacuation of hematoma or extraction of fractured bone. Beyond therapeutic indications, spiritual and hierarchical reasons have been discussed. The Egyptians believed that "evil spirits" would be withdrawn from the subjects during this procedure. In addition, the idea of trephination was the rejoining of ethereal spirit to the body in Peru [5, 6]. Diversity in the array of trephination tools,

A. Pour-Rashidi, J. Aarabi (eds.), *The Principles of Successful Awake Craniotomy*,
https://doi.org/10.1007/978-981-99-2985-6_1

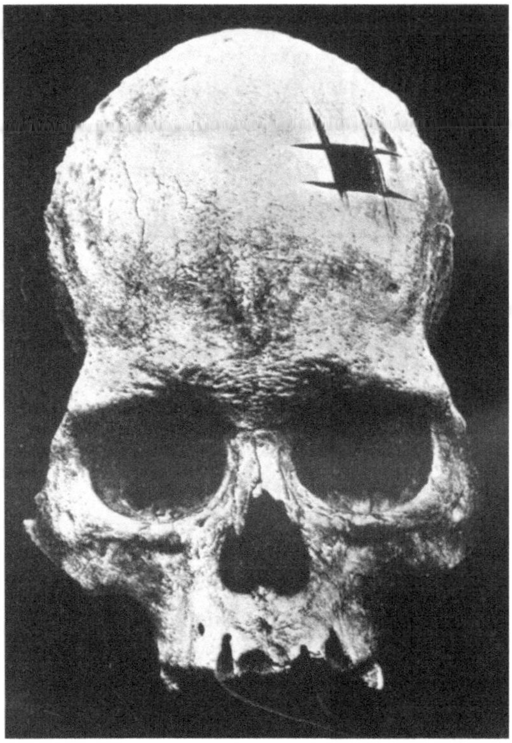

Fig. 1 Anterior aspect of Peruvian "Inca skull", indicating rectangular trephination. (The image was originally published in Squier, E. G., 1877. Peru: Incidents of Travel and Exploration in the Land of the Incas, Henry Holt, New York and reprinted from A Hole in the Head: More Tales in the History of Neuroscience by Charles G. Gross, courtesy of The MIT Press)

hemostasis methods, infection-prevention strategies and training courses are detailed elsewhere and are beyond the scope of this book. Overall, it is not possible to pursue these ancient efforts with modern awake craniotomy; however, tracking its tenets, brain mapping and awake neuroanesthesia/analgesia can provide insight into the progress that resulted in this neurosurgical art.

While available traces of functional localization and surgical analgesia in the ancient era are lacking, the remaining evidence should be considered. Overall, brain localization and dura opening were not targeted in these trephination trainings. Although there was no way of modern brain mapping during ancient trephination, mankind's curiosity has been on a continuous journey. Historical review indicates that available coherent written documents about the growing concentration on modern neuroanatomy originated from the Galenic influence on anatomic teaching. This improved slightly until the end of the medieval era in Europe through Leonardo da Vinci's schematic drawings and markedly strengthened ever since. Hippocrates' impression in neuroanatomy and related ideas can be regarded as a leading step toward later medieval concepts. Hippocrates of Cos (460–377 BC), father of medicine, contributed to The Golden Age of Pericles significantly by developing intellectual medicine including neurosurgery.

Although little is known about his personal life, his legacy as Hippocratic Corpus was recorded by himself or by the aid of his students. Based on observational analysis, Hippocrates provided the first of its kind, a neurosurgical doctrine in his book, "*On Injuries of the Head*" which included neuroanatomical scopes and trephination procedures [7]. Concerning the important aspects of his belief, it was *encephalocentrism* that relied on the executive nature of the brain and later influenced Herophilus and Galen's ideas [8]. This was a revolutionary moment in the history of neuroanatomy, aside from cardiocentrism of Aristotle, and greatly influenced later perspectives in this field. Also, some pre-Hippocratic literature, such as *Iliad* of Homer, discussed neurological significance of traumatic injuries to the nervous system [9]. As such, several areas of the brain such as the center of consciousness have been discussed in *Iliad* of Homer. Apart from these coherent writings, inconsistent records from ancient times refer to neuroanatomy and functional localization. Perhaps the oldest found neurological examination note and assignment of aphasia, paresis and ophthalmoplegia to the traumatic brain injury belongs to Edwin Smith Papyrus from 1600 BC [10]. Albeit some Arabic commentaries and abstract illustrations precede these dates [11, 12].

Performing trephination on patients while being awake was not an unusual or remarkable representation for prehistoric observers, since practical anesthesia was not available until the nineteenth century. Moreover, anesthesia was considered undesirable for a long time until Cappadocia, an ancient Greek physician in the second half of the second century AD. He noted that awake trephination as proper training and *the habit of such persons renders them tolerant of pains and their goodness of spirits and good hopes render them strong in endurance* [13] (Fig. 2). Local anesthesia, narcotics, hallucinogens and alcoholic drink were used on occasion for neurosurgical purposes. Local anesthetics in early trephinations could be herbal preparation of marijuana leaves or Erythroxylum Coca. Coca was chewed by the patient to induce sedative effects and indifference to the pain, although in some regions of ancient Peru, surgeons expelled the smashed leaves onto the field of trephination as a local anesthetic [14, 15]. Ancient Chinese used marijuana leaves in order to prepare local anesthetic for cranial openings and even buried them next to the body of an expired patient [4]. Alcohol has been accepted as an anesthetic since antiquity. Hippocrates used alcoholic immersed tools for its narcotic properties. Peruvian and African surgeons also prescribed alcoholic beverages before trephination. Datura is a shrub whose leaves and flowers are potent anesthetic herbal medicine [16]. The narcotic and hallucinogenic nature of Datura make it an interesting herbal preparation for anesthetists throughout the history of surgery [5].

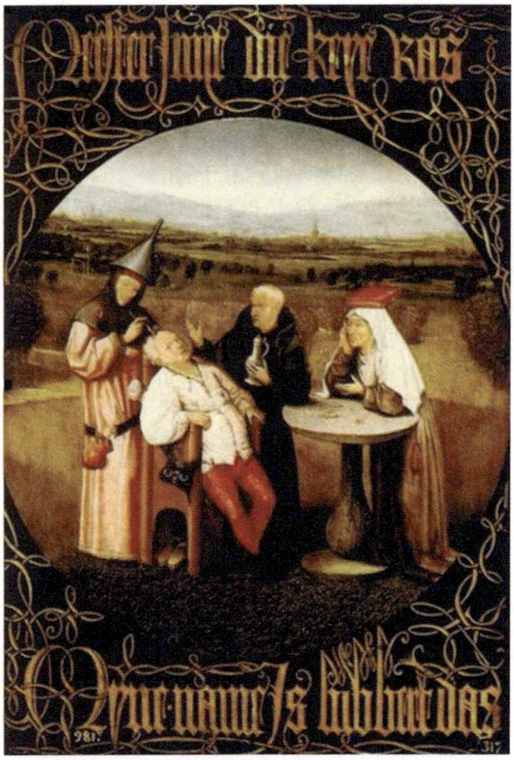

Fig. 2 An illustration attributed to Hieronymus Bosch, 1450–1516 showing awake trephination with assistance of alcoholic drink as an anesthetic agent (License Number: 5466490884627)

Overall, the prehistoric era with its limited findings remains a conundrum involving sporadic and symbolic signs without any commentaries. However, we should explore the foundation of our knowledge base to better augment present practice or redirect misleading deviations.

3 Delineation of Brain Structures and Evolving Functional Neuroanatomy and Neuropsychology

Awake surgery could not be accomplished independent of brain mapping (either positive or negative) and peri-operative neuropsychological testing. These adjuncts date as far back as the history of neurosurgery and never disjoined from its tenets. Although modern intraoperative brain mapping and advanced neuropsychology are now distinct entities, both have a common relationship with functional localization. Since William Osler (1849–1919) in 1916 affixed neurology to psychology, neuropsychology then became a framework to study human behavior in response to nervous system disorders [17]. This later spread to other contemporary scholars, one of which, Karl Lashley (1890–1958) became the figure to bolster this field. Currently, neuropsychological researchers work in proximity with neurosurgery to assess lateralization and localize brain lesions with associative neurobehavioral consequences. Migration from the prehistoric era to modern functional localization embodies fundamental revolution in concepts that construct our current image of brain mapping.

Declaration of encephalocentrism in Hippocratic Corpus can be regarded as the birth of neuroscience by identifying a superior function of the brain, although cardiocentric-encephalocentric opposition lasted about 2000 years in ancient Greece. Still, earlier anatomical surveys of neuronal structure can be regarded in the pre-Hippocratic period without any functional apperception [12]. This concept should be also considered beyond ancient Egyptian observation of lateralizing traumatic brain signs, without the idea of an interconnected central (nervous) system [10].

Galen of Pergamon (129–216 AD), a Greek physician, discovered cell theory and discussed brain ventricles as the center of sensorimotor control and the modulator of consciousness, in accordance with encephalocentric viewpoint. Each ventricle was considered as a critical component that contained the inner senses such as imagination and memory. Specifically, Galen described that the pneuma within the ventricle was responsible for psychological activity and its release caused animals to lose function. While this idea about Galen's cell doctrine created doubt, pneumatic theory seemed logical. Still, the post-Galenic millennium gave rise to cell doctrine in the following centuries in medieval Europe and Persia [18].

Scientific knowledge during the ancient era had been earned and transferred through observation as well as animal dissections executed by Galen. Later, Nemesius of Emesa (fourth century Syrian physician), expanded Galenic thoughts on ventricular theory and introduced functional localization, perhaps through observation of cognitive changes in battlefield injuries [19]. He applied reasoning to distinct functions for each ventricle in his text *On the Nature of Man* which was in parallel with theories of fourth-century medical writer Posidonius of Byzantium. The next centuries were contemporaneous to historical communications between Persian and Greek scientists. In this regard, Arabic translations of Galen and succedent scholars significantly impacted medieval Persian physicians, Ibn Sina (980–1037 AD) and al-Razi (865–935 AD). Ibn Sina, or "Avicenna" in the Latin tradition, declared cell doctrine in *Kitab al-najat* and attributed different mental faculties for distinct ventricles. Similarly, al-Razi described ventricular theory in his book *Al-Mansuri* and even cited Galen for his opinions [18].

During the late medieval age Andreas Vesalius (1514–1564 AD) called Galenic thoughts into question, although he did not suggest a substitutional theory [20]. These doubts continued to establish the basis of modern functional neuroanatomy in relation to brain substance, instead of 1000-year leading ventricular doctrine. This modernization and description of cerebrospinal fluid within ventricles further initiated a transition from ventricles to brain parenchyma illustrated by Leonardo da Vinci (1472–1519 AD) in his drawings. Further contribution in the description of brain surface with gray and white matter featured by Archangelo Piccolomini (1526–1586) concluded the theory of ventricular functional localization.

Beyond the bounds of encephalocentrism, equipotentiality and localization for higher brain functions became the leading confronting challenge between the sixteenth and eighteenth centuries [21]. Pierre Flourens (1794–1867), founder of field theory, like his later counterparts believed in the integration of brain functions and equipotential activity in brain hemispheres. His ideas were concomitant to philosophical assumptions and his unpaired experiments on extirpated animals proved this. Thomas Willis (1621–1675) and Franz Joseph Gall (1758–1828) had identified functions to distinct brain locations; however, their ideas were thought to be a fallacy of orthodox equipotentiality. As it was called the *century of illumination*, growing evidence in the eighteenth century from Gall phrenology theory to Charles Bell's (1774–1829) discovery of decussation of pyramids threw light upon localization legacy [22]. Ultimately, it was Paul Broca (1824–1880) that believed in localization and represented unequivocal evidence by autopsy of an aphasic patient in supporting frontal speech area. It should be noted that Broca's doctrine was completely different from Gall's phrenology and apparently opposed Flourens' equipotentiality.

In the nineteenth century, succeeding contribution of physiologists and anatomists resulted in worldwide development of modern brain functional localization. As such, Joseph Jules Dejerine (1849–1917) (in French) and Carl Wernicke (1848–1905) (in German) participated in localization of language area other than what Broca had named [23]. At the same time, the study of epilepsy reproduced important information in the field of localization that could be highlighted in works of John Hughlings Jackson (1835–1911).

4 Advanced Awake Craniotomy: A Perspective of Brain Mapping and Neuroanesthesia

Contemporary awake craniotomy largely relied on advancement in intraoperative neuromonitoring and modern anesthetic approaches (Fig. 3). This progress led to a fundamental proposal of awake craniotomy as a standard procedure for supratentorial low-grade glioma in patients with high performance scores, although this idea received some criticism [24]. Awake craniotomy indications are widening in essence, from vascular brain surgery to deep brain stimulation. Undoubtedly, it is critical to mention its tenets, track progress and to overcome missteps in this field.

In searching for principles of intraoperative brain mapping, the first step was to consider the nervous system as an electrical excitable organ. In Germany, in 1870, Gustav Fritsch, anatomist, and Eduard Hitzig, neurologist, were the first to excite an animal brain with anterior cortical placing of platinum plates [25]. Their experiment indicated cross-laterality of cortical function and became an introduction to prospective electric cortical mapping. David Ferrier (1843–1928), a nineteenth-century neuropsychologist, became interested in Fritsch and Hitzig's experiments and conducted more delicate animal studies using Faradic current, where complex and sustained movements stimulating paracentral gyri emerged [26]. The culmination of brain mapping studies representing localized cortical function in detail are attributed to the research of Charles Scott Sherrington and Albert Grünbaum on 28 nonhuman primates and observation of more than 400 movements [27].

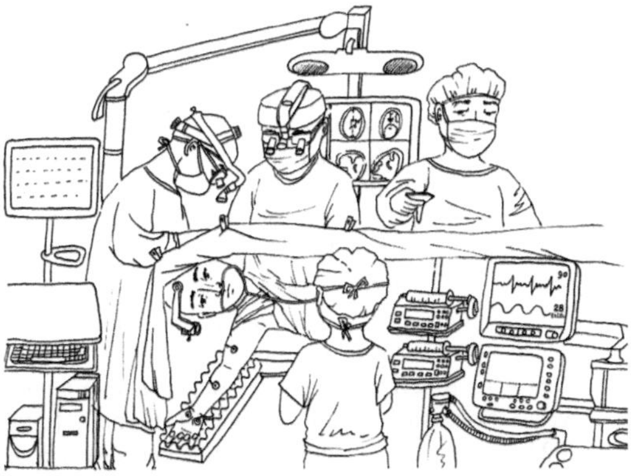

Fig. 3 Modern awake craniotomy operation room with neuromonitoring add-ons (License Number: 5466500206744)

Routine contemporary anesthesia encountered technical obstacles which encouraged further development in functional localization. Enlightenment in human electrical brain mapping has been connected to neuroanesthesia development regarding prevention of intraoperative seizures with concurrent preservation of cortical excitability. The first brain mapping in humans has been attributed to Robert Bartholow (1831–1904) in a case study of cortical stimulation without anesthesia. This was based on the concept of cortical excitability from prior animal experiments of Ferrier, Fritsch and Hitzig. Bartholow and his controversial experiments on the exposed brain of Mary Rafferty confirmed previous animal studies in human brain. His experiments were more precise than prior practices, because he used a unique "electrical room" generated by faradic and galvanic currents with various designated needle electrodes and adjustable voltage [28]. Apart from this specific case, the following human studies were associated with neuroanesthesia development.

Of note, opium and alcohol narcosis were the main anesthetic agents in the early nineteenth century. In the mid-1900s, nitrous oxide, ether and chloroform were practiced in surgical operations; although, it took several decades to implement these anesthetics in neurosurgery. Accordingly, Victor Horsley (1857–1916), a British doctor, performed a series of cortical stimulation in animals and humans about 10 years following Bartholow's experiments [29, 30]. His surgical removal of epileptic focus on 13 consecutive epilepsy patients in 1886 and 1887 was done under chloroform and morphine sedation with durotomy using cocaine, which was introduced by Koller in 1884, as local anesthesia. This may be the first awake epilepsy surgery under direct cortical stimulation. Horsley contributed to "Special Chloroform Committee" in 1901 to delineate safe anesthetic administration. Fedor Krause (1857–1937), a German neurosurgeon, later reproduced Horsley's findings on 142 patients, using only chloroform as an anesthetic agent, with somatotopic mapping of the motor cortex [31].

Wilder Penfield (1891–1976) and his organized intraoperative language mapping was the first major advance in awake craniotomy. His promotion in interactable epilepsy treatment was adopted from his mentor, Otfrid Foerster and pioneered by Feodor Krause. Foerster conducted intraoperative neurophysiologic studies during epilepsy surgeries and localized focal resection. Penfield's experiences under Foerster's mentorship along with Krause's progress in cortical mapping led to an exceptional opportunity for him to build a systematic implantation in awake craniotomy [32]. Penfield's homunculi in several cortical and subcortical regions were reproduced in later studies. Advances in intraoperative neuropsychological and neurophysiological tests as well as development of adaptable methods in neuroanesthesia continued in the late twentieth century. George Ojemann, neurosurgeon at the University of Washington School of Medicine, expanded Penfield's language maps in the 1970s with collaboration of Mitchel S. Berger, to systemized intraoperative neuropsychological testing and application of biphasic stimulation current [33]. Further progress in neuroanesthesia in relation to awake craniotomy can be discussed in either local or general anesthetics.

In the early 1960s, a combination of neuroleptic agents (e.g., droperidol) and opioids (e.g., fentanyl) was recommended to provide amnesia concomitant with anesthesia [34]. This induction of neuroleptanesthesia enabled patients to become easily arousable during surgery to follow commands. Contemporary various derivates of cocaine, including procaine and bupivacaine, were also introduced for long-lasting local anesthesia. Modern awake craniotomies from the 1990s mostly relied on ultrashort-acting opioids (e.g., remifentanil) in combination with propofol due to its favorable pharmacokinetics and anticonvulsive nature [35]. Recent advances in functional neuroimaging revealed functional networks and connectomes with interrelated activities instead of pure modular hypothesis of functional areas [36].

5 Conclusion

Progress from ancient trephination to modern awake craniotomy consisted of inevitable controversies that had to be overcome. Importantly, the challenge for scientific development was impacted by uneven access to experimental resources and accumulated knowledge throughout historical precedence. Induced neuroplasticity around brain lesions is the intriguing context of functional networks. Considering neuroplasticity, staged glioma surgery and transcranial magnetic stimulation-induced functional reorganization are novel headings, which will shape the future of awake craniotomy.

References

1. Michael Apuzzo. The neurosurgeon's toolbox: from stone age to space age. World Neurosurg. 2011. europepmc.org [Internet]. [cited 2022 Jan 21]. https://europepmc.org/article/med/21492638.
2. Furnas D, et al. Traditional craniotomies of the Kisii tribe of Kenya. Ann Plast Surg. 1985. europepmc.org [Internet]. [cited 2022 Jan 21]. https://europepmc.org/article/med/3880206.
3. Broca P. Trépanation chez les Incas. Bulletins et Mémoires de la Société d'Anthropologie de Paris. 1867. persee.fr [Internet]. [cited 2022 Jan 22]. https://www.persee.fr/doc/bmsap_0301-8644_1867_num_2_1_4320.
4. Hobert L, Binello E. Trepanation in ancient China. World Neurosurg. 2017. Elsevier [Internet]. [cited 2022 Jan 27]. https://www.sciencedirect.com/science/article/pii/S1878875016310397?casa_token=E2MzmROCxhUAAAAA:k6nI_YZvzGvjLhXGF18WTJb4MggvngqxBaIOLY_G--ZO5unnYnX6OGr5OpB2_MWqvNnuR1WaOPA.

5. Rifkinson-Mann S. Cranial surgery in ancient Peru. Neurosurg. 1988. academic.oup.com [Internet]. [cited 2022 Jan 27]. https://academic.oup.com/neurosurgery/article-abstract/23/4/411/2745913.
6. Rutkow IM. Trephination. JAMA Surg. 2000. jamanetwork.com [Internet]. [cited 2022 Jan 27]. https://jamanetwork.com/journals/jamasurgery/article-abstract/390709.
7. Missios S. Hippocrates, Galen, and the uses of trepanation in the ancient classical world. Neurosurg Focus. 2007. thejns.org [Internet]. [cited 2022 Jan 28]. https://thejns.org/focus/view/journals/neurosurg-focus/23/1/foc-07_07_e11.xml.
8. Pearce JMS. The neuroanatomy of Herophilus. Eur Neurol. 2013. karger.com [Internet]. [cited 2022 Jan 28]. https://www.karger.com/Article/Abstract/346232.
9. Sahlas DJ. Functional neuroanatomy in the pre-Hippocratic era: observations from the Iliad of Homer. Neurosurgery. 2001. academic.oup.com [Internet]. [cited 2022 Jan 23]. https://academic.oup.com/neurosurgery/article-abstract/48/6/1352/3773580.
10. Kamp MA, Tahsim-Oglou Y, Steiger HJ, Hänggi D. Traumatic brain injuries in the ancient Egypt: insights from the Edwin Smith Papyrus. J Neurol Surgery A Cent Eur Neurosurg. 2012;73(4):230–7.
11. Frank M. History and bibliography of anatomic illustration. 1920 [cited 2022 Jan 23]. https://unthsc-ir.tdl.org/handle/20.500.12503/25865.
12. Herrlinger R. History of medical illustration,... 1979. [Internet]. [cited 2022 Jan 23]. https://scholar.google.com/scholar?hl=en&as_sdt=0%2C5&q=Herrlinger%2C+R.+%281979%29.+%22History+of+Medical+Illustration%2C+from+Antiquity+to+1600%22&btnG=.
13. Adams F. The extant works of aretaeus: the cappadocian [Internet]. 1856 [cited 2022 Jan 27]. https://books.google.com/books?hl=en&lr=&id=XCMwAAAAYAAJ&oi=fnd&pg=PR1&dq=+Extant+Works+of+Aretaues,+the+Cappadocian.+&ots=B2SC7f-RB1&sig=yrisV27NPa70m_s1-OprbTUe4cg.
14. Frost EA. A history of neuroanesthesia. The Wondrous Story of Anesthesia. 2014:871–85. https://link.springer.com/chapter/10.1007/978-1-4614-8441-7_64
15. Froeschner EH. Historical vignette two examples of ancient skull surgery. J Neurosurg. 1992;76:550–2.
16. Monira KM, Munan SM. Review on datura metel: a potential medicinal plant. Glob J Res Med Plants Indig Med GJRMI [Internet]. 2012 [cited 2022 Jan 29];1(4):123–32. www.gjrmi.comwww.gjrmi.com.
17. Bogousslavsky J, Boller F, Iwata M. A history of neuropsychology [Internet]. 2019 [cited 2022 Jan 31]. https://books.google.com/books?hl=en&lr=&id=3rSXDwAAQBAJ&oi=fnd&pg=PP1&dq=neuropsychology+history&ots=QAvkFLqMxe&sig=QvIaTzvuu2K9kJfFYF2MNmbd_f4.
18. Green CD. Where did the ventricular localization of mental faculties come from? J Hist Behav Sci [Internet]. 2003 Mar [cited 2022 Jan 31];39(2):131–42. www.interscience.wiley.com.
19. Perspectives. [cited 2022 Jan 31]. www.thelancet.com.
20. Rose FC. Cerebral localization in antiquity. J Hist Neurosci. 2009;18(3):239–47.
21. Tizard B.. Theories of brain localization from Flourens to Lashley. Med Hist. 1959. cambridge.org [Internet]. 2022 [cited 2022 Feb 1]. https://www.cambridge.org/core/journals/medical-history/article/theories-of-brain-localization-from-flourens-to-lashley/8EEAE1727AF3A785D22D131D318A524A.
22. Sabbatini RME. Phrenology: the history of brain localization. 1997. academia.edu [Internet]. [cited 2022 Feb 1]. https://www.academia.edu/download/50321734/Phrenology_the_history_of_Brain_Localiza20161115-9407-1huidqg.pdf.
23. Folzenlogen Z, Ormond DR. A brief history of cortical functional localization and its relevance to neurosurgery. Neurosurg Focus. 2019. thejns.org [Internet]. [cited 2022 Feb 1]. https://thejns.org/focus/view/journals/neurosurg-focus/47/3/article-pE2.xml.
24. Duffau H. Is non-awake surgery for supratentorial adult low-grade glioma treatment still feasible? Neurosurg Rev. 2018;41(1):133–9.
25. Fritsch G, Hitzig E. Uber die elektrische Erregbarkeit des Grosshirns. 1870. ci.nii.ac.jp [Internet]. [cited 2022 Feb 1]. https://ci.nii.ac.jp/naid/10008144995/.
26. Ferrier D. The functions of the brain. London: Smith [Internet]. [cited 2022 Feb 1]. https://scholar.google.com/scholar?hl=en&as_sdt=0%2C5&q=Ferrier+D%3A+The+Functions+of+the+Brain.+London%3A+Smith%2C+Elder%2C+%26+Co%2C+1876&btnG=.
27. Griinbaum DASF, Sherrington CS. Observations on the physiology of the cerebral cortex of some of the higher apes. (Preliminary communication.). Proc R Soc London [Internet]. 1902 Apr 4 [cited 2022 Feb 1];69(451–458):206–9. https://royalsocietypublishing.org/.
28. Patra D, Hess R, Abi-Aad K, et al. Roberts Bartholow: the progenitor of human cortical stimulation and his contentious experiment. Neurosurg Fous. 2019. thejns.org [Internet]. [cited 2022 Feb 1]. https://thejns.org/focus/view/journals/neurosurg-focus/47/3/article-pE6.xml.
29. Horsley V. Remarks on ten consecutive cases of operations upon the brain and cranial cavity to illustrate the details and safety of the method employed. Br Med J. 1887. ncbi.nlm.nih.gov [Internet]. [cited 2022 Feb 1]. https://www.ncbi.nlm.nih.gov/pmc/articles/pmc2534542/.
30. Horsley V.. Brain-surgery. Br Med J. 1886. JSTOR [Internet]. [cited 2022 Feb 1]. https://www.jstor.org/stable/25269252.
31. Krause F. Surgery of the brain and spinal cord: based on personal experiences [Internet]. 1912 [cited 2022 Feb 1]. https://books.google.com/books?hl=en&lr=&id=QvkSAAAAYAAJ&oi=fnd&pg=PA273&dq=Krause+F:+Surgery+of+the+Brain+and+Spinal+Cord+Based+on+Personal+Experiences.+New+York:+Rebman+Co,+1912&ots=SZ-7XnVbpl&sig=a9jeIL3xK3RSnFHt7nm6VCaHCmk.

32. Snyder P, Whitaker HA. Neurologic heuristics and artistic whimsy: the cerebral cartography of Wilder Penfield. J Hist Neurosci. 2013. Taylor Fr [Internet]. 2013 Jul 1 [cited 2022 Feb 1];22(3):277–91. https://www.tandfonline.com/doi/abs/10.1080/0964704X.2012.757965.
33. Berger M, Kincaid J, Ojemann G, Lettich E. Brain mapping techniques to maximize resection, safety, and seizure control in children with brain tumors. Neurosurgery. 1989. academic.oup.com [Internet]. [cited 2022 Feb 1]. https://academic.oup.com/neurosurgery/article-abstract/25/5/786/2748951.
34. Bulsara K, Johnson J, Villavicencio AT. Improvements in brain tumor surgery: the modern history of awake craniotomies. Neurosurg Focus. 2005. Citeseer [Internet]. [cited 2022 Feb 1]. https://citeseerx.ist.psu.edu/viewdoc/download?doi=10.1.1.631.4500&rep=rep1&type=pdf.
35. Rahimpour S, Haglund MM, Friedman AH, Duffau H. History of awake mapping and speech and language localization: from modules to networks. Neurosurg Focus. 2019. thejns.org [Internet]. [cited 2022 Feb 1]. https://thejns.org/focus/view/journals/neurosurg-focus/47/3/article-pE4.xml.
36. Mapping critical cortical hubs and white matter pathways by direct electrical stimulation: an original functional atlas of the human brain. Elsevier [Internet]. [cited 2022 Feb 2]. https://www.sciencedirect.com/science/article/pii/S1053811919308286.

Awake Craniotomy for Tumor Surgery <Awake Craniotomy, Tumor, Mapping>

Amin Tavallaii and Alireza Mansouri

1 Introduction

Despite advances in the field of surgical neuro-oncology, optimal surgical management of brain tumors located within or near eloquent areas is challenging for neurosurgeons. In these circumstances, there are two main goals of surgery: a) maximal tumor resection to improve tumor control and survival, and b) preservation of preoperative neurological functions to improve the patient's quality of life. There is a body of evidence supporting the significant role of maximal resection in increasing overall survival and reduction of recurrence rate following surgical management of intrinsic brain tumors especially gliomas (either low-grade or high-grade) [1–21]. Much effort has been done to achieve an ideal balance between these two goals and awake craniotomy (AC) is one of the most known and appreciated techniques in this regard.

The first applications of AC were in the field of epilepsy surgery. In the 1990s, George Ojemann and Mitchel Berger developed this technique for resection of brain tumors intending to reduce postoperative neurological deficits. This technique was applied to patients with eloquent areas lesions for minimizing the permanent neurological deficits together with increasing the extent of the resection [22]. Later on, Hugues, Duffau, and his colleagues revised this technique to achieve maximal safe resection of intrinsic brain tumors [23].

Currently, AC with or without intraoperative monitoring has become a well-known, feasible, and standard option for surgical management of brain tumors, especially gliomas located near eloquent areas [24]. Awake surgery enables the surgical team to have a continuous and almost real-time evaluation of the patient's neurological functioning during resection. Application of intraoperative electrical stimulation may also help in more precise localization of speech and sensorimotor functional areas with cessation or initiation of the patient's respective responses [25, 26].

There is a growing body of evidence emphasizing the superiority of AC over resection under general anesthesia (GA) in terms of the higher extent of resection and greater postoperative preservation of neurological functions following resection of tumors located within or near eloquent areas responsible for motor or speech functions [10, 27, 28]. Implementation of AC in the field of neuro-oncology has led to the safe and

A. Tavallaii (✉)
Department of Pediatric Neurosurgery,
Akbar Childrens Hospital, Mashhad University of Medical Sciences, Mashhad, Iran
e-mail: tavallaeia@mums.ac.ir

A. Mansouri
Department of Neurosurgery, Penn State Hershey Medical Center, Penn State University, Hershey, PA, USA
e-mail: amansouri@pennstatehealth.psu.edu

A. Pour-Rashidi, J. Aarabi (eds.), *The Principles of Successful Awake Craniotomy*,
https://doi.org/10.1007/978-981-99-2985-6_2

successful resection of many lesions which were previously considered "inoperable" [29]. The application of this technique is not limited to glioma surgery and has facilitated a development toward the management of other neuro-oncological entities such as brain metastasis.

Throughout this chapter, we present a clear perspective concerning the role of AC in the surgical management of brain tumors by covering topics such as indications and patient selection, technical nuances, and possible morbidities. Among various indications for AC, our focus will be the application of this technique in the safe resection of gliomas, although we point out other neuro-oncological entities as well. The available intraoperative adjuncts and mapping tools as well as localization methods for various functional areas during awake surgery has also been reviewed.

2 Indications and Patient Selection

Like the management of many other entities in neurosurgery, patient selection plays a pivotal role in the determination of surgical success and postoperative clinical outcomes. Patients who are selected for AC must meet a list of specific requirements to be considered good candidates for this technique. As it can be drawn from the nature of AC, the main application of this surgical technique in neuro-oncology should be the resection of brain tumors involving or located within proximity of eloquent areas. A substantial proportion of these tumors had been previously dealt with as inoperable tumors [30, 31].

Despite the significant role of pre-operative mapping techniques such as functional MRI (fMRI), diffusion tensor imaging (DTI), and magneto-encephalography (MEG) in preoperative planning, these modalities lack sufficient accuracy to rule out the eloquent nature of a specific region of interest [32–34]. For example, despite the acceptable reliability of these modalities in lateralizing speech-related areas, they are not sufficient for accurate delineation of the boundaries of these functional areas [35, 36]. Therefore, the absence of tumor extension to the functional areas identified in preoperative mapping techniques does not necessarily obviate the need for AC, and the decision to proceed with awake or asleep surgery should be sought considering these shortcomings. Moreover, the intraoperative displacement of anatomical structures following craniotomy and resection of large brain tumors renders neuronavigation-based localization techniques unreliable and they should not be considered an appropriate alternative for AC [34]. The application of AC is more emphasized in cases with potential concern about the involvement of functional areas responsible for speech, and these cases significantly benefit from real-time intraoperative monitoring of verbal functioning during mapping. However, for tumors located within the proximity of sensorimotor cortices, resection under GA may also result in favorable neurological outcomes [37].

Emotional and psychological conditions affecting patient cooperation, present and possible neurological deficits, history, and frequency of seizures are crucial in the process of finding the best candidates for AC. There are few absolute contraindications for AC such as patients with aphasia, severe/long-lasting motor deficit, cognitive disabilities (or mental disabilities), dementia, and significant behavioral disorders impairing optimal patient cooperation during surgery [38]. Risk factors and comorbidities such as morbid obesity (BMI > 40), history of obstructive apnea, smoking, and gastroesophageal reflux are considered relative, rather than absolute, contraindications. Strategies such as the use of laryngeal mask airways (LMA) before and after intraoperative mapping, and pre-operative prescription of cough suppressants and anti-reflux medications are among the approaches to address such challenges [26, 37, 39]. Psychological disorders such as emotional lability and anxiety are not contraindications of AC if proven to be completely treated and the disorder is in the stable phase based on preoperative psychological testing. Although this is a challenging topic and remains controversial, a history of seizures may raise concern about the incidence of intraoperative seizures; however, iced Ringer's solution or iced saline and IV propofol could be used in case it occurs. Patients with any radiological evidence pointing to an impending herniation (i.e., midline shift of more than 2 cm) on preoperative imaging studies are at greater risk for mass effect exacerbation during patient awakening and AC is relatively contraindicated for them. Nonetheless, if the surgeon opts to pursue with AC in such patients, initial internal debulking of safer tumor zones (away from eloquent areas) before patient awakening can be used as a feasible approach. We will briefly provide an overview of some of the specific pathologies that AC technique can be considered as a potential option in their management.

3 Glioma

Gliomas are the most common primary brain tumor and comprise a heterogeneous group of infiltrative glial neoplasms classified based on histologic and molecular characteristics. These tumors account for about 30% of all brain tumors and 80% of malignant ones [40]. Gliomas mostly involve and infiltrate the white matter tracts responsible for connecting different functional areas. This infiltrative nature significantly limits the feasibility of achieving complete surgical resection. Moreover, in high-grade gliomas (HGGs) (i.e., GBM), the aggressive behavior of the tumor and its limited response to adjuvant therapies such as chemotherapy and radiation therapy, strikingly increase the recurrence rate and mortality to an extent that results in a 15-month median overall survival (OS) [16, 18, 41–44]. Nevertheless, surgical resection has proven to be the most effective treatment modality and an independent prognostic factor in the management of these tumors.

Surgical resection of gliomas located within or near eloquent areas responsible for speech, motor, cognition, and other functions (i.e., Broca's and Wernicke's areas, motor cortices or pathways, etc.) may accompany significant postoperative neurological deficits and morbidities. Furthermore, when considering low-grade glioma (LGG), multiple reports indicate that eloquent areas or pathways may be displaced by tumors or undergo different kinds of reorganization due to neuroplasticity [45–47]. This structural and functional reorganization highlights the challenges in the resection of these tumors and emphasizes the necessity of using intraoperative mapping techniques. Various intraoperative adjuncts are introduced to overcome such challenges, and AC is one of the most interesting ones implemented alone or in combination with other techniques which will be discussed further in this chapter. The reported extent of resection and functional outcomes of patients with either LGG or HGG operated on using AC have been promising. Moreover, the combination of AC with intraoperative stimulation has led to improved resection and a significant reduction in postoperative neurological deficits in multiple studies [48–53].

These challenges in glioma resection and the remarkable ability of AC to improve the extent of resection and clinical outcome have made it the most suitable indication for AC. However, the introduction of new imaging and mapping techniques and the existence of few reports of suboptimal results following AC in glioma resection have cast doubt on the applications of this modality. In the most recent attempt to reduce this uncertainty, researchers performed qualitative data synthesis on the results of existing studies and concluded that AC is still the best available technique to achieve maximal safe resection and it can be considered as a gold standard [24].

3.1 Low-Grade Glioma (LGG)

LGGs are slow-growing lesions that grow along the white matter tracts and have the potential to undergo malignant transformation [54]. These lesions may be asymptomatic or present with nonspecific symptoms, seizures, and less commonly with neurological deficits. The asymptomatic nature of these lesions is consistent with their slow growth, which allows some kinds of neural plasticity.

The management of LGGs is challenging but there are multiple strategies to control the challenges [55–72]. Although this controversy is less pronounced while dealing with symptomatic LGGs located in non-eloquent areas, and the recommendations in these cases are more for maximal resection, the main challenge will be the optimal approach to LGGs located in eloquent areas [64, 66, 68, 69, 73–77]. In this case, various recommendations spanning from a conservative approach and close patient follow-up to maximal and aggressive surgical resection can be found in the literature [55, 57, 59, 64, 66, 71, 78–85]. However, the rule about the effect of the extent of resection on the outcomes of gliomas also applies to LGGs, and surgical resection can lead to a significant increase in patients' 5-year OS [54, 82, 86–90]. There is also evidence demonstrating a positive effect of early surgical resection of LGGs which affects the tumor control interval, progression-free survival, and overall survival [91, 92]. Early surgical resection has other advantages such as reducing the rate of seizures as well as decreasing the risk of malignant transformation in these tumors [64, 68, 75, 77, 82, 83, 88, 93–95]. Interestingly, in LGGs, even the term "supramaximal resection" has been suggested, which includes the resection of a grossly normal margin around the tumor, and some evidence supports the improvement of clinical outcomes following this technique [64, 73, 77].

However, there are concerns about postoperative deficits following surgical resection of these tumors and, in particular, significant concerns about behavioral and neurocognitive disorders following surgery have been mentioned [61, 96]. Given the significant life expectancy of these patients, which is reported to be around 14 to 15 years, maintaining the quality of life and reducing postoperative neurological deficits is of significant importance and AC can play a key role in achieving this goal [82, 86]. In this regard, there is evidence to support the positive effect of AC and intraoperative cortical mapping on increasing the extent of resection, improving the OS, and reducing postoperative neurological deficits, which will be discussed in detail later [29, 97, 98]. In contrast, the potential for neuroplasticity is much less appreciated at the subcortical level than in the cortical areas [99, 100]. Therefore, resection of the cortical areas involved by LGG may not cause significant neurological morbidities, but damage to the subcortical pathways may cause irreversible neurological deficits [101, 102]. Ultimately, using a real-time monitoring and mapping technique such as AC can benefit both cortical and subcortical areas.

3.2 High-Grade Glioma (HGG)

HGGs, especially glioblastoma (GBM), are the most common primary brain tumors. Unfortunately, despite multi-modality treatments, these tumors have an unfavorable prognosis and continue to be a therapeutic challenge in the field of neuro-oncology. The efficacy of existing treatment modalities, which are a combination of maximal resection and adjuvant chemotherapy and radiotherapy, is limited and despite these treatments, the median life expectancy of patients with GBM is around 15 months and their 5-year OS is approximately 6.8% [41–44].

In HGGs, like other gliomas, the extent of resection is the most important known prognostic factor [9, 18, 103, 104]. Unfortunately, the role of AC in the management of HGGs has not been well studied, compared to LGGs, and outcomes are not well documented. For example, few studies have focused on the clinical outcome of AC in GBM, most of which are retrospective observational studies or systematic reviews consisting of a mixed population of patients managed by awake and asleep craniotomies, and no randomized controlled trial can be found in this field [10, 29]. The results of these studies will be discussed in the outcomes section of this chapter.

The resection of tumors located in the insular area, the vast majority of which are gliomas, is one of the significant challenges in the field of neuro-oncology. The insula is involved in a range of sensory, cognitive, limbic, and language processing functions and has numerous connections to important functional areas such as the amygdala, thalamus, cingulate, orbitofrontal, and sensory cortices [105–108]. This area is also surrounded by important parts of the motor and language pathways [109]. In addition, the basal ganglia and internal capsule are adjacent to the medial insula. The presence of blood vessels feeding these eloquent areas around the insula also adds to the anatomical complexity of this region and the difficulty of resecting tumors located within, and any surgical approach to this area should be performed diligently.

Gliomas in this area, despite the highly eloquent nature of the insula, are more likely to present with seizures, and presentation with mild neurological deficits are less common [110, 111]. Therefore, efforts for maximal resection of insular tumors, despite the improvement of OS may worsen neurological functioning in patients with minor preoperative neurological deficits. The natural history of insular gliomas is not very predictable but the positive effect of the extent of resection on 5-year OS has been well demonstrated. Considering the selection bias in the existing studies, resection of at least 90% of Insular gliomas increased 5-year OS from 84% to 100% in patients with grade II glioma and increased 2-year OS from 75% to 91% in patients with grade III and IV gliomas [110].

One of the most common surgical approaches for resection of insular gliomas is the transcortical approach using intraoperative mapping techniques. In this approach, awake language mapping is used for lesions located in the dominant hemisphere, as well as subcortical motor mapping to determine the location of the internal capsule adjacent to the medial aspect of the tumor [110, 112]. In this approach, the extent of craniotomy depends on the size and location of the tumor, and the decision to perform intraoperative mapping. It should be noted that when planning to perform awake language mapping, a small limited surgical field may confine mapping areas that do not have a language function ("negative") and may not permit determination of functional ("positive") language areas. However, it has been demonstrated that using negative mapping, the possibility of postoperative language deficit is very low, and its incidence has been reported to be approximately 1.6%. Such results indicate the safety of glioma resection in this area based on negative mapping alone and through a limited craniotomy [46]. The use of subcortical mapping also allows the detection and protection of functional pathways around this area [106, 113]. Considering the efficacy of these techniques in various studies, a significant reduction in postoperative neurological complications to 3-9% has been reported following the implementation of advanced mapping techniques [110–112, 114, 115].

4 Metastasis

Brain metastases are one of the common intracranial tumors, and the incidence has been increasing in recent studies [116–119]. The significant effect of surgical resection of these lesions on survival and tumor control has been well demonstrated [120, 121]. However, resection of these tumors in eloquent areas can be associated with significant morbidities. Despite the general belief in the non-infiltrative nature of brain metastases, there is increasing evidence of a degree of infiltration in the surrounding normal tissue by metastatic tumoral cells [122–125]. The significance of this issue becomes more apparent during the surgical approach to metastatic tumors located in eloquent areas. In such cases, AC can be a suitable treatment option like the approach to primary brain tumors. Therefore, the role of AC in the resection of metastatic intracranial lesions is evolving. In the most recent study in this field, a systematic review consisting of 7 studies and 104 patients who underwent metastasis resection using the AC technique reported a gross total resection (GTR) rate of 61% and postoperative neurological complications rate of 27%. However, these complications have been mostly short-term and 96% of patients with neurological complications have had excellent postoperative recovery [126]. Permanent neurological deficits have been reported in only 1% of all these patients, and most of them were due to brain edema, ischemia, vascular insult, or iatrogenic damage to the white matter tracts [126, 127]. These results are even more favorable than those of gliomas operated on with AC and indicate the safety of this technique in the management of patients with brain metastases.

Alternative approaches to brain metastases located in eloquent areas are stereotactic radiosurgery (SRS) and conventional radiotherapy, with a recurrence rate of 46–76% for these treatment modalities compared to a recurrence rate of 9% in patients operated on with the AC technique [126, 128, 129]. Therefore, higher efficacy is one of the other advantages of using AC in the resection of brain metastases located in eloquent areas.

5 Technical Nuances

Successful implementation of the AC technique depends on the formation of a team collaboration between the various groups involved, such as the surgical team, anesthesiologists, and the team responsible for patient assessment during the awake phase. Ideally, this cooperation should begin before surgery and at the patient selection stage and continue until after surgery and management of possible complications.

The role of the anesthesiologist is very important in the preoperative stage to evaluate the patient's comorbidities and determine the patient's suitability for surgery under AC as well as during the operation. Preventing the patient from becoming agitated and moving unexpectedly is a very sensitive task of the anesthesia team during AC which can prevent injury to the patient, contamination of the surgical field, and impaired accuracy of intraoperative adjuncts.

Communication between surgeon and patient can also play an important role in reducing patient anxiety during surgery. A clear and sufficient description of the procedure, the process, and the symptoms that the patient may experience in the awake phase should be provided to them. Reassuring the patient that all necessary measures are being taken to control the pain and discomfort during surgery can lead to a significant reduction in stress and anxiety. Also, in cases where there is a concern about high levels of patient stress, starting anxiolytic medications on the day of admission can help with the situation.

Before the surgery, intraoperative tasks and assessments (i.e., language and/or motor) to be performed during the awake phase will be practiced with the patient to familiarize him/her with these tasks. The most complex intraoperative assessments are related to language function, which are more time-consuming and more difficult than motor-related assessments. This is largely due to the multiplicity and heterogeneity of areas responsible for language. In these language-related assessments, various tasks such as naming and narration are used to localize responsible eloquent areas [130]. Therefore, the patient's familiarity with these tasks requires more practice prior to surgery.

During surgery, the patient is usually placed in a position that maintains comfort during the awake phase, provides a clear field of vision for the patient, and enables interaction with anesthesia and assessment teams. This is necessary so that the patient can view images, provide feedbacks, and execute commands during surgery. Such conditions are best met in the semi-lateral position. Other advantages of the semi-lateral position include better airway preservation and providing optimal surgical orientation to the perisylvian and motor cortex areas. In cases where it is necessary to use a Mayfield head holder for immobilization (e.g., when neuronavigation is required), it is best to first inject a local anesthetic agent such as bupivacaine at the pin sites and place the Mayfield after a few minutes. In most patients, anticonvulsant prophylaxis, mannitol, and dexamethasone are given at the beginning of surgery as a standard step to prevent intraoperative seizures and reduce cerebral edema. Preoperative antiemetics also help with reducing the incidence of nausea and vomiting during the awake phase. Maintaining a body temperature above 36 °C is important, especially during the mapping stage.

The most common AC technique is known as the awake-asleep-awake (AAA) technique. In this procedure, the patient is first intubated and anesthesized under GA. In the initial asleep phase, a craniotomy is performed with a technique similar to surgery under GA. The patient is then awakened and undergoes intraoperative mapping and resection of the tumor within eloquent areas, and then enters the final asleep phase to complete the surgery [131]. A variety of anesthesia regimens and techniques are introduced such as using local anesthesia and nerve blocks during the awake phase and IV sedation with drugs (e.g., propofol, fentanyl, or dexmedetomidine) during the asleep phase, which are discussed in detail in chapter "Principles of Neuroanesthesia for Awake Craniotomy".

Manipulation of the dura can be painful and may cause patient agitation during the awake phase. Therefore, it is recommended that the dura-opening be performed before the patient awakens and after the injection of local anesthetics around the middle meningeal artery. The assessment team continuously monitors the patient's sensorimotor and language functioning during mapping and resection, and the frequency of these assessments will increase when the surgeon is concerned about getting close to the eloquent areas. Gogos et al. (2020) introduced the "triple motor mapping" technique for resection of such tumors under GA, which includes "transcranial and/or direct cortical stimulation for monitoring during resection, monopolar stimulation for cortical mapping, and monopolar and bipolar stimulation for subcortical mapping" [37].

The method and content of assessments and tests are determined depending on the patient's hand dominance status and the side and location of the tumor. After mapping, light sedation can be used during resection to increase the patient's comfort, but many surgeons prefer to perform the tumor resection in a fully awake patient and under constant monitoring of the patient's functioning to be able to perform subcortical mapping during resection. It is preferable to perform surgical resection with the aid of intraoperative adjuncts such as a Cavitron UltraSonic Aspirator (CUSA) and the least usage of electrocoagulation. Safe resection requires being at least 1–2 cm away from the areas marked as positive during cortical mapping [132]. Also, subpial dissection and avoidance of vascular manipulation can prevent tissue hypoperfusion and ischemia [133, 134]. In cases where a new neurological deficit is observed during assessments, the resection should be stopped immediately and then continue with the resection conditionally (preferably from areas farther away from that area) if the new deficit is completely resolved within less than 5 min.

6 Intraoperative Adjuncts

Numerous surgical adjuncts are available to improve clinical outcomes following AC. These adjuncts may help with the localization of cortical and subcortical functional areas using various tasks in the awake phase, like intraoperative mapping with or without direct electrical stimulation (DES); or they may aid surgeons with maintaining surgical orientation during resection and increasing the extent of tumor resection such as intraoperative MRI (iMRI), ultrasound and neuronavigation. For example, tasks such as object naming can be useful in locating eloquent language-related areas with accuracy to prevent the occurrence or exacerbation of aphasia after surgery [135]. Also, subcortical mapping using electrical stimulation can be useful in the detection and protection of white matter tracts associated with eloquent cortical areas [113]. The significant role of subcortical mapping in reducing the postoperative rate of motor and language-related neurological deficits has been demonstrated in several studies [113, 136–138]. Confirmation of achieving surgical goals and maximal tumor resection by intraoperative imaging modalities such as iMRI are other advantages of using intraoperative surgical adjuncts [139–142]. However, there is a contradiction about the extent of these methods' ability to achieve those goals and are discussed further in the following section.

6.1 Intraoperative Mapping Techniques

Currently available intraoperative mapping techniques are the result of the efforts of Foster, Penfield, and Cushing, which have also entered the field of neuro-oncology in recent decades [12,

135, 136, 143–145]. The general purpose of these techniques is to prepare an accurate functional map of the cortical and subcortical eloquent areas as well as real-time monitoring of these areas to avoid damage to them during tumor resection [146]. Mapping during the awake phase is used for the localization of areas involved in language, vision, and cognitive functions; however, eloquent areas related to sensorimotor functions can be localized in both awake and asleep phases [28, 31, 147, 148].

DES, being the most common intraoperative mapping technique, involves stimulating the exposed cortical surface and/or subcortical area within the surgical field using a weak electrical current. To do this, the test area is divided into small areas at a distance of 1 cm from each other and each area is stimulated up to three non-consecutive times [26]. The response caused by this stimulation, as a result of the depolarization, will vary depending on the function of the stimulated eloquent region. If the stimulus is applied to the area related to the language function, it causes that area to temporarily stop functioning and cause immediate transient disruption of the patient's speech, which to some extent mimics the postoperative neurological deficit that will follow the resection of that area. However, if the motor cortex is stimulated, there will be an evidence of induction of function in the form of involuntary motor response and the sensation of muscle contractions by the awake patient, or electromyographic evidence of muscle contractions during the asleep phase [23, 149–151]. A bipolar stimulator is commonly used for stimulation with 60Hz electrical pulses starting at 1 mA and gradually increasing until the desired response is achieved. It should be noted that none of the cortical points be stimulated twice in a row. The intensity of the electric current used in different studies varied from 2 to 10mA and durations of up to 4s are recommended for the stimulation [23, 152–154]. Speech impairment usually occurs up to a current of 2–3mA and there is no need to increase the current beyond that for mapping the areas responsible for speech. Mapping the motor cortex in an asleep patient may require 10mA of electrical current. However, the use of currents higher than 4mA in awake patients is associated with an increased risk of intraoperative seizures. Therefore, continuous electrocorticography (ECoG) should be performed during mapping to detect after-discharges and in case of detecting any, the surgical field should be rinsed with iced Ringer's solution. After complete resolution of the discharge, the surgeon can proceed with the stimulation using a current intensity of at least 1mA less than before. It has been observed that the rate of intraoperative seizures is significantly higher while using a monopolar instead of a bipolar stimulator [155]. Subcortical mapping is mostly used to determine the proximity of the tumor to the corticospinal tract, and it has led to a higher GTR rate [156, 157].

Existing data show that DES is a safe technique and is well tolerated by patients if certain precautions are met [26, 158, 159]. Various reasons such as optimal sensitivity and low false-negative rate, interrogation of both cortical and subcortical pathways, and high efficacy in detecting language-related areas have made this technique one of the most attractive adjuncts used during AC. Therefore, DES is considered the gold standard for intraoperative mapping during AC [29, 113, 160]. Similarly, the results of a meta-analysis indicate a less than 4% rate of permanent neurological deficit following tumor resection with the aid of intraoperative DES [29]. Simultaneous use of continuous motor-evoked potential (MEP) can also increase the accuracy and safety of resection of tumors located within the proximity of motor areas [147, 150, 161]. Intraoperative mapping techniques are constantly evolving. In addition, recent innovations such as passive cortical mapping have been introduced in which ECoG is used to identify responsible functional areas while performing verbal, motor, and cognitive tasks. By obviating the need for stimulation, this technique can reduce potential complications such as intraoperative seizures and shorten the duration of surgery. Of course, the application of this technique is still under investigation, and it is hoped that soon it will be a viable alternative, when DES may not be safe [162, 163].

6.2 Intraoperative MRI

The use of a method that can accurately determine tumor remnants during surgery and reduce the distorting effect of resection-induced brain shift on the accuracy of landmarks has been an unattainable goal before the introduction of iMRI. However, currently, iMRI and intraoperative mapping have formed an ideal and available armamentarium for maximal safe resection of either HGGs or LGGs. The integration of structural findings from iMRI with functional findings from mapping methods has helped to improve the resection results of intrinsic brain lesions and is now accepted as a standard for surgical management in many well-equipped centers [164, 165]. Other MRI-related modalities can also be performed intraoperatively and can provide the surgeon with more valuable information for a safe resection.

The outcomes of using iMRI were inconsistent in terms of affecting the extent of resection [166]. However, the results of recent studies are more supporting the significant effect of this modality on increasing the extent of glioma resection (either high-grade or low-grade) [50, 104, 167–171]. The benefits of iMRI also include reducing postoperative neurological deficits and improving the quality of life in patients with tumors involving eloquent areas [172]. Tuominen et al. (2013) have shown that the combination of iMRI and AC with DES was more effective in reducing the rate of postoperative neurological complications following resection of gliomas located in eloquent areas related to speech and motor compared to the use of iMRI alone during resection under GA [169]. In another study, a comparison of patients undergoing AC surgery with and without iMRI indicated a greater need for reoperation in patients who were operated on without iMRI [173]. Two retrospective studies have investigated the effect of iMRI on the resection of insular gliomas under AC, with similar results in support of the positive effect of this modality on the extent of resection and reduction of the rate of permanent postoperative neurological deficits [174, 175].

Despite these advantages, the use of iMRI during AC may result in longer surgery and requires more cooperation from the awake patient. Some studies have raised concerns about the impact of prolonged surgery on the incidence of surgical infection and complications such as deep venous thrombosis (DVT), but the use of iMRI does not appear to have increased the rate of these complications [132, 176].

6.3 Intraoperative Ultrasound (IOUS)

Ultrasound is another intraoperative adjunct which guides the surgeon toward maximal safe resection, particularly in glioma surgery. This technology was has been used since before the iMRI, and it is more available, cheaper, and safer than the other modalities. Surgeons can use the intraoperative ultrasound (IOUS) for opening the dura, appropriate corticectomy, and differentiating the normal tissues from the tumor as well as determining the tumoral margins which may result in a higher extent of tumor resection. The greatest advantage of the IOUS is that it guides the surgeon step by step without being interrupted by the brain shift. Nevertheless, the IOUS is an operator-dependent technology which can be a potential limitation [130].

6.4 Fluorescence-Guided Surgery (FGS)

Fluorescence-guided surgery (FGS) was explored during the last two decades based on the light-emission reflected by radiation-absorbed substances. Currently, 5-aminolevulinic acid (5-ALA) is widely prescribed orally, then its emission is received intraoperatively via the microscope equipped with specific optical filters about 4–6h after ingestion which shows the tumor in red in its center and pinkish in the marginal areas. This method is more useful in resection of HGGs and malignant tumors [120].

7 Complications and Morbidities

Although many studies have addressed the effectiveness of AC, the possible side effects and morbidities of this technique have been less studied and discussed [177]. Therefore, in this section, a comprehensive discussion is presented about intraoperative and postoperative morbidities, as well as an appropriate approach to the prevention and management of complications.

In a study of 25 cases who underwent AC for resection of intrinsic tumors, the rate of complications during and after surgery was 92% and 68%, respectively, which seems to be significant. The most common complications during surgery include hypertension possibly due to pain and psychological stress, agitation and discomfort, pain, seizures, and tachycardia, in a decreasing order of prevalence [178–182]. These morbidities are generally related either to the surgical technique or to the factors related to anesthesia.

The most common complications associated with the surgical technique are intraoperative seizures and the development of new neurological deficits. Intraoperative seizure is one of the most stressful complications during AC. The prevalence of intraoperative seizure among patients who had undergone awake surgery for glioma has been reported to be about 8% in a systematic review of 25 relevant studies [183]. This rate may be higher in tumors located in certain anatomical areas such as supplementary motor area and insula [178, 184, 185]. Moreover, most of these seizures occur following the use of stimulation-based mapping methods, especially 50Hz and train-of-five techniques [186]. The occurrence of intraoperative seizures is significant in that they can lead to AC failure and its premature termination, thereby reducing the extent of tumor resection as well as increasing the likelihood of postoperative transient neurological deficits [26, 184, 187, 188]. Currently, the most recommended approach to seizures during AC includes using iced Ringer solution on the cortical surface and in case it fails in cessation of seizures, the administration of intravenous propofol. However, preventive measures such as preoperative prophylactic use of anticonvulsants and their continuation until surgery and administration of an intraoperative booster dose before craniotomy have reduced the incidence of this complication to 0.5% [26]. Furthermore, both monopolar and bipolar stimulators for intraoperative brain mapping are available and corticospinal fibers are more sensitive to the monopolar stimulators. Also, motor cortex can be better identified by the monopolar probe compared to using the bipolar stimulator [186].

The incidence of permanent neurological deficits after AC is significantly low [189]. The most common new postoperative neurological deficits are related to speech, among which approximately 1.5% are permanent. Sanai et al. (2008) reported 22% and 1.6% rates for the transient and permanent postoperative language deficits, respectively [46]. The prevalence of motor neurological deficits and their likelihood of becoming permanent is lower than that of language deficits, which is probably due to the lower need for AC in the resection of tumors only involving motor areas compared to tumors involving areas responsible for speech, and this is in addition to the fact that language network is more complex, involving numerous different subcortical pathways and cortical hubs [31, 190]. Preservation of motor function following AC is largely predicted by the preservation of intraoperative normal motor function and lack of any evidence of ischemia on postoperative MRI [31, 191]. Prompt initiation of motor and/or speech rehabilitation is of great importance for patients with postoperative neurological deficits and should be started as soon as possible [192].

Incidents such as apnea, airway obstruction, and insufficient ventilation, as well as agitation and poor patient cooperation, are among the complications associated with anesthesia. Impaired airway patency is one of the major concerns in AC patients (especially during the awake phase) which can also have adverse effects on surgical resection by causing hypercapnia and exacerbating cerebral edema. This event is more common in obese patients and patients who are overly sedated. Using tools such as LMA can better protect the airway in such patients. Also, balancing the desired level of sedation with the awakeness required during AC through appropriate anesthesia regimen helps maintain the patient's respiratory drive at an optimal level. In this regard, the results of using anesthesia regimen containing Dexmedetomidine in maintaining the desired level of sedation and patient cooperation, as well as preventing the occurrence of respiratory events have been promising [26, 193].

As with any other surgical technique, a precise preoperative assessment including the patient's medical comorbidities, the frequency of preoperative seizures, the state of neurological function, as well as the patient's level of cooperation and anxiety significantly helps with appropriate patient selection, taking preventive precautions to reduce complications and being prepared to deal with them in case of occurrence.

8 Efficacy and Outcome

The general impression is that AC can be a safe and effective approach to increase the extent of resection and improve outcomes in patients with tumors within eloquent areas of the brain, and the majority of existing studies report approximately 90% resection rate and more than 50% GTR achievement using this technique [194].

Despite the attractiveness of the AC technique, few studies have compared the results of this technique with craniotomy under GA. Among them, the findings of an observational study by Eseonu et al. (2017) are interesting with higher GTR rate and postoperative KPS score, and shorter hospital stay following resection of gliomas located within the motor area using AC technique compared to resection under GA [28]. The results of a systematic review and meta-analysis performed on this subject showed that in 2351 cases of gliomas located in the motor area (either LGG or HGG), the extent of resection was significantly higher with the AC technique compared to surgery under GA [195]. However, in the results of an older systemic review that examined the clinical outcome of 1037 patients with gliomas located within the eloquent area, similar clinical outcomes were reported for AC and GA [196]. In a recent meta-analysis consisting of 10 studies and 833 patients, the AC technique without DES had similar results to GA in terms of neurological outcomes, while the use of DES during AC resulted in more favorable neurological outcomes, a higher extent of resection, and shorter hospital stay compared to GA [197]. Therefore, it seems that AC with intraoperative DES can be considered a gold standard in this field [29].

In terms of the effect of the AC technique on patient survival, Duffau et al. (2005) reported an OS rate of 91% for patients who underwent LGG resection using the AC technique compared to a 57% rate for the GA group [198]. Contrary to these results, the study of Gravesteijn et al. (2018) failed to show the superiority of either AC technique or resection under GA in terms of 1–5 years survival [199]. A comparison of these two techniques in terms of recurrence rate and PFS has also had conflicting and ambiguous results. In a study by Eseonu et al. (2017), similar recurrence rates were reported for AC technique and resection under GA, but in another study, Martino et al. (2013) reported a PFS rate of 5.7 years for the AC technique versus 3.7 years for resection under GA [28, 200]. Regarding these results, mindful awareness should be exercised about the molecular profiling of the tumors and the types of adjuvant therapies while interpreting them.

Glioma grades can be considered as one of the important factors influencing the outcome because LGGs generally show a different infiltrative nature compared to HGGs [1]. This difference can lead to variations in the effectiveness of AC in LGGs and HGGs [48]. Few studies have focused on AC outcomes in HGGs such as GBM, and most of the studies on AC in patients with glioma have been performed on a mixed population of LGGs and HGGs, or exclusively on LGGs. Clinical outcomes in this regard are associated with more controversy. In a retrospective study, Gerritsen et al. (2019) specifically published data on the use of AC in the management of patients with GBM, which has shown a higher resection rate and lower postoperative complications in the AC group despite the lack of survival benefit [201]. In a systematic review consisting of this study and 13 other retrospective studies, the lack of a positive effect of the AC technique on survival in 278 patients with GBM was confirmed. Also, in this study, the rate of GTR achievement and occurence of early and late postoperative complications following the use of AC technique were reported to be 74.7%, 34.5%, and 1.9%, respectively [189]. Due to the scarcity of studies in this field, the effect of increasing the extent of resection using AC on the survival of GBM patients is still controversial.

It seems that despite numerous review studies on the clinical outcomes of AC and its comparison with the results of tumor resection under GA and the reporting of promising results for AC, there are still contradictions and controversies regarding the superiority of AC in terms of its potential to improve survival rate and long-term clinical outcomes. These contrasts are even more pronounced in the case of HGGs. It seems that most of these disagreements are due to the small sample size, heterogeneity of the study populations, differences in outcome measures used, and the retrospective nature of the vast majority of existing studies. Therefore, there is a serious need to design and implement larger high-quality prospective studies in this field.

9 Conclusion

The AC technique is one of the most well-known and attractive methods for resection of tumors located in eloquent areas, which after decades of its introduction has been continuously refined to improve its outcomes. With these improvements, particularly in the field of intraoperative mapping, many of the barriers to safe resection of these tumors have been largely removed and further resection has been made possible by protecting the cortical areas and subcortical pathways responsible for neurological functions. However, the available information in this area still has significant ambiguities, the resolution of which depends on future prospective comparative studies.

References

1. Berger MS, Deliganis AV, Dobbins J, Keles GE. The effect of extent of resection on recurrence in patients with low grade cerebral hemisphere gliomas. Cancer. 1994;74(6):1784–91.
2. Martin C, Alexander E, Wong T, Schwartz R, Jolesz F, Black PM. Surgical treatment of low-grade gliomas in the intraoperative magnetic resonance imager. Neurosurg Focus. 1998;4(4):E10.
3. Berger MS, Rostomily RC. Low grade gliomas: functional mapping resection strategies, extent of resection, and outcome. J Neurooncol. 1997;34(1):85–101.
4. Laws ER, Parney IF, Huang W, Anderson F, Morris AM, Asher A, et al. Survival following surgery and prognostic factors for recently diagnosed malignant glioma: data from the Glioma Outcomes Project. J Neurosurg. 2003;99(3):467–73.
5. Sanai N, Berger MS. Glioma extent of resection and its impact on patient outcome. Neurosurgery. 2008;62(4):753–64; discussion 264–6.
6. Aghi MK, Nahed BV, Sloan AE, Ryken TC, Kalkanis SN, Olson JJ. The role of surgery in the management of patients with diffuse low grade glioma: a systematic review and evidence-based clinical practice guideline. J Neurooncol. 2015;125(3):503–30.
7. D'Amico RS, Englander ZK, Canoll P, Bruce JN. Extent of resection in glioma-a review of the cutting edge. World Neurosurg. 2017;103:538–49.
8. Brown TJ, Brennan MC, Li M, Church EW, Brandmeir NJ, Rakszawski KL, et al. Association of the extent of resection with survival in glioblastoma: a systematic review and meta-analysis. JAMA Oncol. 2016;2(11):1460–9.
9. Chaichana KL, Jusue-Torres I, Navarro-Ramirez R, Raza SM, Pascual-Gallego M, Ibrahim A, et al. Establishing percent resection and residual volume thresholds affecting survival and recurrence for patients with newly diagnosed intracranial glioblastoma. Neuro Oncol. 2014;16(1):113–22.
10. Gerritsen JKW, Arends L, Klimek M, Dirven CMF, Vincent AJE. Impact of intraoperative stimulation mapping on high-grade glioma surgery outcome: a meta-analysis. Acta Neurochir. 2019;161(1):99–107.
11. McGirt MJ, Mukherjee D, Chaichana KL, Than KD, Weingart JD, Quinones-Hinojosa A. Association of surgically acquired motor and language deficits on overall survival after resection of glioblastoma multiforme. Neurosurgery. 2009;65(3):463–9; discussion 469–70.
12. Sanai N, Berger MS. Intraoperative stimulation techniques for functional pathway preservation and glioma resection. Neurosurg Focus. 2010;28(2):E1.
13. Keles GE, Anderson B, Berger MS. The effect of extent of resection on time to tumor progression and survival in patients with glioblastoma multiforme of the cerebral hemisphere. Surg Neurol. 1999;52(4):371–9.
14. Keles GE, Chang EF, Lamborn KR, Tihan T, Chang C-J, Chang SM, et al. Volumetric extent of resection and residual contrast enhancement on initial surgery as predictors of outcome in adult patients with hemispheric anaplastic astrocytoma. J Neurosurg. 2006;105(1):34–40.
15. McGirt MJ, Chaichana KL, Gathinji M, Attenello FJ, Than K, Olivi A, et al. Independent association of extent of resection with survival in patients

with malignant brain astrocytoma: clinical article. J Neurosurg. 2009;110(1):156–62.
16. Lacroix M, Abi-Said D, Fourney DR, Gokaslan ZL, Shi W, DeMonte F, et al. A multivariate analysis of 416 patients with glioblastoma multiforme: prognosis, extent of resection, and survival. J Neurosurg. 2001;95(2):190–8.
17. Lamborn KR, Chang SM, Prados MD. Prognostic factors for survival of patients with glioblastoma: Recursive partitioning analysis. Neuro Oncol. 2004;6(3):227–35.
18. Sanai N, Polley M-Y, McDermott MW, Parsa AT, Berger MS. An extent of resection threshold for newly diagnosed glioblastomas: clinical article. J Neurosurg. 2011;115(1):3–8.
19. Smith JS, Chang EF, Lamborn KR, Chang SM, Prados MD, Cha S, et al. Role of extent of resection in the long-term outcome of low-grade hemispheric gliomas. J Clin Oncol. 2008;26(8):1338–45.
20. Vecht CJ, Avezaat CJ, van Putten WL, Eijkenboom WM, Stefanko SZ. The influence of the extent of surgery on the neurological function and survival in malignant glioma. A retrospective analysis in 243 patients. J Neurol Neurosurg Psychiatry. 1990;53(6):466.
21. Ushio Y, Kochi M, Hamada J-i, Kai Y, Nakamura H. Effect of surgical removal on survival and quality of life in patients with supratentorial glioblastoma. Neurol Med Chir. 2005;45(9):454–61.
22. Surbeck W, Hildebrandt G, Duffau H. The evolution of brain surgery on awake patients. Acta Neurochir. 2015;157(1):77–84.
23. Duffau H. Surgery of low-grade gliomas: towards a 'functional neurooncology'. Curr Opin Oncol. 2009;21(6):543–9.
24. Foster CH, Morone PJ, Cohen-Gadol A. Awake craniotomy in glioma surgery: is it necessary? J Neurosurg Sci. 2019;63(2):162–78.
25. Berger MS. Functional mapping-guided resection of low-grade gliomas. Clin Neurosurg. 1995;42:437–52.
26. Hervey-Jumper SL, Li J, Lau D, Molinaro AM, Perry DW, Meng L, et al. Awake craniotomy to maximize glioma resection: methods and technical nuances over a 27-year period. J Neurosurg. 2015;123(2):325–39.
27. Hervey-Jumper SL, Berger MS. Maximizing safe resection of low- and high-grade glioma. J Neurooncol. 2016;130(2):269–82.
28. Eseonu CI, Rincon-Torroella J, ReFaey K, Lee YM, Nangiana J, Vivas-Buitrago T, et al. Awake craniotomy vs craniotomy under general anesthesia for perirolandic gliomas: evaluating perioperative complications and extent of resection. Neurosurgery. 2017;81(3):481–9.
29. De Witt Hamer PC, Robles SG, Zwinderman AH, Duffau H, Berger MS. Impact of intraoperative stimulation brain mapping on glioma surgery outcome: a meta-analysis. J Clin Oncol. 2012;30(20):2559–65.
30. Han SJ, Morshed RA, Troncon I, Jordan KM, Henry RG, Hervey-Jumper SL, et al. Subcortical stimulation mapping of descending motor pathways for perirolandic gliomas: assessment of morbidity and functional outcome in 702 cases. J Neurosurg. 2018;131(1):201–8.
31. Magill ST, Han SJ, Li J, Berger MS. Resection of primary motor cortex tumors: feasibility and surgical outcomes. J Neurosurg. 2018;129(4):961–72.
32. Tarapore PE, Tate MC, Findlay AM, Honma SM, Mizuiri D, Berger MS, et al. Preoperative multimodal motor mapping: a comparison of magnetoencephalography imaging, navigated transcranial magnetic stimulation, and direct cortical stimulation. J Neurosurg. 2012;117(2):354–62.
33. Wu JS, Zhou LF, Tang WJ, Mao Y, Hu J, Song YY, et al. Clinical evaluation and follow-up outcome of diffusion tensor imaging-based functional neuronavigation: a prospective, controlled study in patients with gliomas involving pyramidal tracts. Neurosurgery. 2007;61(5):935–48; discussion 948-9.
34. Nimsky C, Ganslandt O, Hastreiter P, Wang R, Benner T, Sorensen AG, et al. Intraoperative diffusion-tensor MR imaging: shifting of white matter tracts during neurosurgical procedures—initial experience. Radiology. 2005;234(1):218–25.
35. Tarapore PE, Chang EF, Gabriel R, Berger MS, Nagarajan SS. Magnetoencephalographic imaging for neurosurgery. In: Pillai JJ, editor. Functional brain tumor imaging. New York, Springer; 2014. p. 111–28.
36. Spena G, Nava A, Cassini F, Pepoli A, Bruno M, D'Agata F, et al. Preoperative and intraoperative brain mapping for the resection of eloquent-area tumors. A prospective analysis of methodology, correlation, and usefulness based on clinical outcomes. Acta Neurochir. 2010;152(11):1835–46.
37. Gogos AJ, Young JS, Morshed RA, Hervey-Jumper SL, Berger MS. Awake glioma surgery: t echnical evolution and nuances. J Neurooncol. 2020;147(3):515–24.
38. Nabavi A, Goebel S, Doerner L, Warneke N, Ulmer S, Mehdorn M. Awake craniotomy and intraoperative magnetic resonance imaging: patient selection, preparation, and technique. Top Magn Reson Imaging. 2008;19(4):191–6.
39. Leuthardt EC, Lim CC, Shah MN, Evans JA, Rich KM, Dacey RG, et al. Use of movable high-field-strength intraoperative magnetic resonance imaging with awake craniotomies for resection of gliomas: preliminary experience. Neurosurgery. 2011;69(1):194–205; discussion 206.
40. Goodenberger ML, Jenkins RB. Genetics of adult glioma. Cancer Genet. 2012;205(12):613–21.
41. Ostrom QT, Cioffi G, Gittleman H, Patil N, Waite K, Kruchko C, et al. CBTRUS statistical report: primary brain and other central nervous system tumors diagnosed in the United States in 2012-2016. Neuro Oncol. 2019;21(Suppl 5):v1–v100.

42. Wen PY, Kesari S. Malignant gliomas in adults. N Engl J Med. 2008;359(5):492–507.
43. Stupp R, Mason WP, van den Bent MJ, Weller M, Fisher B, Taphoorn MJ, et al. Radiotherapy plus concomitant and adjuvant temozolomide for glioblastoma. N Engl J Med. 2005;352(10):987–96.
44. Behin A, Hoang-Xuan K, Carpentier AF, Delattre JY. Primary brain tumours in adults. Lancet (London, England). 2003;361(9354):323–31.
45. Duffau H, Capelle L, Denvil D, Sichez N, Gatignol P, Lopes M, et al. Functional recovery after surgical resection of low grade gliomas in eloquent brain: hypothesis of brain compensation. J Neurol Neurosurg Psychiatry. 2003;74(7):901–7.
46. Sanai N, Mirzadeh Z, Berger MS. Functional outcome after language mapping for glioma resection. N Engl J Med. 2008;358(1):18–27.
47. Thulborn KR, Carpenter PA, Just MA. Plasticity of language-related brain function during recovery from stroke. Stroke. 1999;30(4):749–54.
48. Gupta DK, Chandra PS, Ojha BK, Sharma BS, Mahapatra AK, Mehta VS. Awake craniotomy versus surgery under general anesthesia for resection of intrinsic lesions of eloquent cortex--a prospective randomised study. Clin Neurol Neurosurg. 2007;109(4):335–43.
49. Sacko O, Lauwers-Cances V, Brauge D, Sesay M, Brenner A, Roux FE. Awake craniotomy vs surgery under general anesthesia for resection of supratentorial lesions. Neurosurgery. 2011;68(5):1192–8; discussion 1198–9.
50. Peruzzi P, Bergese SD, Viloria A, Puente EG, Abdel-Rasoul M, Chiocca EA. A retrospective cohort-matched comparison of conscious sedation versus general anesthesia for supratentorial glioma resection. Clinical article. J Neurosurg. 2011;114(3):633–9.
51. Tsitlakidis A, Foroglou N, Venetis CA, Patsalas I, Hatzisotiriou A, Selviaridis P. Biopsy versus resection in the management of malignant gliomas: a systematic review and meta-analysis: a review. J Neurosurg. 2010;112(5):1020–32.
52. Whittle IR, Pringle A-M, Taylor R. Effects of resective surgery for left-sided intracranial tumours on language function: a prospective study. Lancet. 1998;351(9108):1014–8.
53. McGirt MJ, Chaichana KL, Attenello FJ, Weingart JD, Than K, Burger PC, et al. Extent of surgical resection is independently associated with survival in patients with hemispheric infiltrating low-grade gliomas. Neurosurgery. 2008;63(4):700–7. author reply 7-8
54. Duffau H. Diffuse low-grade gliomas in adults. New York: Springer; 2017.
55. McKhann GM, Duffau H. Low-grade glioma: epidemiology, pathophysiology, clinical features, and treatment. Neurosurg Clin N Am. 2019;30(1):xiii–xiv.
56. Diwanji TP, Engelman A, Snider JW, Mohindra P. Epidemiology, diagnosis, and optimal management of glioma in adolescents and young adults. Adolesc Health Med Ther. 2017;8:99–113.
57. Duffau H. Awake mapping is not an additional surgical technique but an alternative philosophy in the management of low-grade glioma patients. Neurosurg Rev. 2018;41(2):689–91.
58. Darlix A, Mandonnet E, Freyschlag CF, Pinggera D, Forster MT, Voss M, et al. Chemotherapy and diffuse low-grade gliomas: a survey within the European Low-Grade Glioma Network. Neurooncol Pract. 2019;6(4):264–73.
59. Al-Tamimi YZ, Palin MS, Patankar T, MacMullen-Price J, O'Hara DJ, Loughrey C, et al. Low-grade glioma with foci of early transformation does not necessarily require adjuvant therapy after radical surgical resection. World Neurosurg. 2018;110:e346–e54.
60. Corrivetti F, Herbet G, Moritz-Gasser S, Duffau H. Prosopagnosia induced by a left anterior temporal lobectomy following a right temporo-occipital resection in a multicentric diffuse low-grade glioma. World Neurosurg. 2017;97:756.e1–5.
61. Duffau H. Is non-awake surgery for supratentorial adult low-grade glioma treatment still feasible? Neurosurg Rev. 2018;41(1):133–9.
62. Duffau H. Paradoxes of evidence-based medicine in lower-grade glioma: to treat the tumor or the patient? Neurology. 2018;91(14):657–62.
63. Claus EB, Walsh KM, Wiencke JK, Molinaro AM, Wiemels JL, Schildkraut JM, et al. Survival and low-grade glioma: the emergence of genetic information. Neurosurg Focus. 2015;38(1):E6.
64. Duffau H. Long-term outcomes after supratotal resection of diffuse low-grade gliomas: a consecutive series with 11-year follow-up. Acta Neurochir. 2016;158(1):51–8.
65. Hendriks EJ, Idema S, Hervey-Jumper SL, Bernat AL, Zwinderman AH, Barkhof F, et al. Preoperative resectability estimates of nonenhancing glioma by neurosurgeons and a resection probability map. Neurosurgery. 2019;85(2):E304–e13.
66. Jo J, Williams B, Smolkin M, Wintermark M, Shaffrey ME, Lopes MB, et al. Effect of neoadjuvant temozolomide upon volume reduction and resection of diffuse low-grade glioma. J Neurooncol. 2014;120(1):155–61.
67. Picart T, Herbet G, Moritz-Gasser S, Duffau H. Iterative surgical resections of diffuse glioma with awake mapping: how to deal with cortical plasticity and connectomal constraints? Neurosurgery. 2019;85(1):105–16.
68. Picart T, Duffau H. Awake resection of a left operculo-insular low-grade glioma guided by cortico-subcortical mapping. Neurosurg Focus. 2018;45(VideoSuppl2):V1.
69. Still MEH, Roux A, Huberfeld G, Bauchet L, Baron MH, Fontaine D, et al. Extent of resection and residual tumor thresholds for postoperative total seizure freedom in epileptic adult patients harboring a supratentorial diffuse low-grade glioma. Neurosurgery. 2019;85(2):E332–e40.

70. Almairac F, Duffau H, Herbet G. Contralesional macrostructural plasticity of the insular cortex in patients with glioma: a VBM study. Neurology. 2018;91(20):e1902–e8.
71. Vanacôr C, Duffau H. Analysis of legal, cultural, and socioeconomic parameters in low-grade glioma management: variability across countries and implications for awake surgery. World Neurosurg. 2018;120:47–53.
72. Coget A, Deverdun J, Bonafé A, van Dokkum L, Duffau H, Molino F, et al. Transient immediate postoperative homotopic functional disconnectivity in low-grade glioma patients. Neuroimage Clin. 2018;18:656–62.
73. Lima GLO, Dezamis E, Corns R, Rigaux-Viode O, Moritz-Gasser S, Roux A, et al. Surgical resection of incidental diffuse gliomas involving eloquent brain areas. Rationale, functional, epileptological and oncological outcomes. Neurochirurgie. 2017;63(3):250–8.
74. Mirza FA, Shamim MS. Extent of resection and timing of surgery in adult low grade glioma. J Pak Med Assoc. 2017;67(6):959–61.
75. Englot DJ, Han SJ, Berger MS, Barbaro NM, Chang EF. Extent of surgical resection predicts seizure freedom in low-grade temporal lobe brain tumors. Neurosurgery. 2012;70(4):921–8; discussion 928.
76. Jakola AS, Myrmel KS, Kloster R, Torp SH, Lindal S, Unsgård G, et al. Comparison of a strategy favoring early surgical resection vs a strategy favoring watchful waiting in low-grade gliomas. JAMA. 2012;308(18):1881–8.
77. Yordanova YN, Moritz-Gasser S, Duffau H. Awake surgery for WHO Grade II gliomas within "non-eloquent" areas in the left dominant hemisphere: toward a "supratotal" resection. Clinical article. J Neurosurg. 2011;115(2):232–9.
78. Best B, Nguyen HS, Doan NB, Gelsomino M, Shabani S, Ahmadi Jazi G, et al. Gliomas: survival differences between metropolitan and non-metropolitan counties. J Neurosurg Sci. 2019;63(2):114–20.
79. Mandonnet E, Duffau H. An attempt to conceptualize the individual onco-functional balance: why a standardized treatment is an illusion for diffuse low-grade glioma patients. Crit Rev Hematol. 2018;122:83–91.
80. Carpentier A, Chauvet D, Reina V, Beccaria K, Leclerq D, McNichols RJ, et al. MR-guided laser-induced thermal therapy (LITT) for recurrent glioblastomas. Lasers Surg Med. 2012;44(5):361–8.
81. Reijneveld JC, Sitskoorn MM, Klein M, Nuyen J, Taphoorn MJ. Cognitive status and quality of life in patients with suspected versus proven low-grade gliomas. Neurology. 2001;56(5):618–23.
82. Jakola AS, Skjulsvik AJ, Myrmel KS, Sjåvik K, Unsgård G, Torp SH, et al. Surgical resection versus watchful waiting in low-grade gliomas. Ann Oncol. 2017;28(8):1942–8.
83. Tovar-Spinoza Z, Choi H. MRI-guided laser interstitial thermal therapy for the treatment of low-grade gliomas in children: a case-series review, description of the current technologies and perspectives. Childs Nerv Syst. 2016;32(10):1947–56.
84. Sloan AE, Ahluwalia MS, Valerio-Pascua J, Manjila S, Torchia MG, Jones SE, et al. Results of the NeuroBlate System first-in-humans Phase I clinical trial for recurrent glioblastoma: clinical article. J Neurosurg. 2013;118(6):1202–19.
85. Oberheim Bush NA, Chang S. Treatment strategies for low-grade glioma in adults. J Oncol Pract. 2016;12(12):1235–41.
86. Capelle L, Fontaine D, Mandonnet E, Taillandier L, Golmard JL, Bauchet L, et al. Spontaneous and therapeutic prognostic factors in adult hemispheric World Health Organization Grade II gliomas: a series of 1097 cases: clinical article. J Neurosurg. 2013;118(6):1157–68.
87. Duffau H, Taillandier L. New concepts in the management of diffuse low-grade glioma: proposal of a multistage and individualized therapeutic approach. Neuro Oncol. 2015;17(3):332–42.
88. Roelz R, Strohmaier D, Jabbarli R, Kraeutle R, Egger K, Coenen VA, et al. Residual tumor volume as best outcome predictor in low grade glioma - a nine-years near-randomized survey of surgery vs. biopsy. Sci Rep. 2016;6:32286.
89. Sanai N, Berger MS. Operative techniques for gliomas and the value of extent of resection. Neurotherapeutics. 2009;6(3):478–86.
90. Sanai N, Berger MS. Recent surgical management of gliomas. Adv Exp Med Biol. 2012;746:12–25.
91. Lima GL, Duffau H. Is there a risk of seizures in "preventive" awake surgery for incidental diffuse low-grade gliomas? J Neurosurg. 2015;122(6):1397–405.
92. Yordanova YN, Duffau H. Supratotal resection of diffuse gliomas - an overview of its multifaceted implications. Neurochirurgie. 2017;63(3):243–9.
93. Chang EF, Potts MB, Keles GE, Lamborn KR, Chang SM, Barbaro NM, et al. Seizure characteristics and control following resection in 332 patients with low-grade gliomas. J Neurosurg. 2008;108(2):227–35.
94. You G, Huang L, Yang P, Zhang W, Yan W, Wang Y, et al. Clinical and molecular genetic factors affecting postoperative seizure control of 183 Chinese adult patients with low-grade gliomas. Eur J Neurol. 2012;19(2):298–306.
95. Gunnarsson T, Olafsson E, Sighvatsson V, Hannesson B. Surgical treatment of patients with low-grade astrocytomas and medically intractable seizures. Acta Neurol Scand. 2002;105(4):289–92.
96. Klein M, Duffau H, De Witt Hamer PC. Cognition and resective surgery for diffuse infiltrative glioma: an overview. J Neurooncol. 2012;108(2):309–18.
97. De Benedictis A, Moritz-Gasser S, Duffau H. Awake mapping optimizes the extent of resection for low-grade gliomas in eloquent areas. Neurosurgery. 2010;66(6):1074–84; discussion 1084.
98. Chang EF, Clark A, Smith JS, Polley MY, Chang SM, Barbaro NM, et al. Functional mapping-guided resection of low-grade gliomas in eloquent areas

of the brain: improvement of long-term s urvival. Clinical article. J Neurosurg. 2011;114(3):566–73.

99. Duffau H. The huge plastic potential of adult brain and the role of connectomics: new insights provided by serial mappings in glioma surgery. Cortex. 2014;58:325–37.
100. Duffau H. Diffuse low-grade gliomas and neuroplasticity. Diagn Interv Imaging. 2014;95(10):945–55.
101. Ghinda CD, Duffau H. Network plasticity and intraoperative mapping for personalized multimodal management of diffuse low-grade gliomas. Front Surgery. 2017;4:3.
102. Wu CX, Pu S, Lin Y, Wang YZ, Jiang T, Xie J, et al. Fractionated resection on low grade gliomas involving Broca's area and insights to brain plasticity. Chin Med J (Engl). 2008;121(20):2026–30.
103. Chaichana KL, Jusue-Torres I, Lemos AM, Gokaslan A, Cabrera-Aldana EE, Ashary A, et al. The butterfly effect on glioblastoma: is volumetric extent of resection more effective than biopsy for these tumors? J Neurooncol. 2014;120(3):625–34.
104. Senft C, Bink A, Franz K, Vatter H, Gasser T, Seifert V. Intraoperative MRI guidance and extent of resection in glioma surgery: a randomised, controlled trial. Lancet Oncol. 2011;12(11):997–1003.
105. Michaud K, Duffau H. Surgery of insular and paralimbic diffuse low-grade gliomas: technical considerations. J Neurooncol. 2016;130(2):289–98.
106. Hervey-Jumper SL, Berger MS. Insular glioma surgery: an evolution of thought and practice. J Neurosurg. 2019;130(1):9–16.
107. Maffei A, Haley M, Fontanini A. Neural processing of gustatory information in insular circuits. Curr Opin Neurobiol. 2012;22(4):709–16.
108. Augustine JR. Circuitry and functional aspects of the insular lobe in primates including humans. Brain Res Brain Res Rev. 1996;22(3):229–44.
109. Herbet G, Moritz-Gasser S, Duffau H. Direct evidence for the contributive role of the right inferior fronto-occipital fasciculus in non-verbal semantic cognition. Brain Struct Funct. 2017;222(4):1597–610.
110. Sanai N, Polley MY, Berger MS. Insular glioma resection: assessment of patient morbidity, survival, and tumor progression. J Neurosurg. 2010;112(1):1–9.
111. Przybylowski CJ, Baranoski JF, So VM, Wilson J, Sanai N. Surgical morbidity of transsylvian versus transcortical approaches to insular gliomas. J Neurosurg. 2019;132(6):1731–8.
112. Hervey-Jumper SL, Li J, Osorio JA, Lau D, Molinaro AM, Benet A, et al. Surgical assessment of the insula. Part 2: validation of the Berger-Sanai zone classification system for predicting extent of glioma resection. J Neurosurg. 2015;124(2):482–8.
113. Duffau H, Peggy Gatignol ST, Mandonnet E, Capelle L, Taillandier L. Intraoperative subcortical stimulation mapping of language pathways in a consecutive series of 115 patients with Grade II glioma in the left dominant hemisphere. J Neurosurg. 2008;109(3):461–71.
114. Di Carlo DT, Cagnazzo F, Anania Y, Duffau H, Benedetto N, Morganti R, et al. Post-operative morbidity ensuing surgery for insular gliomas: a systematic review and meta-analysis. Neurosurg Rev. 2020;43(3):987–97.
115. Mandonnet E. Transopercular resection of IDH-mutated insular glioma: a critical appraisal of an initial experience. World Neurosurg. 2019;132:e563–e76.
116. Counsell CE, Collie DA, Grant R. Incidence of intracranial tumours in the Lothian region of Scotland, 1989-90. J Neurol Neurosurg Psychiatry. 1996;61(2):143–50.
117. Smedby KE, Brandt L, Bäcklund ML, Blomqvist P. Brain metastases admissions in Sweden between 1987 and 2006. Br J Cancer. 2009;101(11):1919–24.
118. Nayak L, Lee EQ, Wen PY. Epidemiology of brain metastases. Curr Oncol Rep. 2012;14(1):48–54.
119. Walker AE, Robins M, Weinfeld FD. Epidemiology of brain tumors: the national survey of i ntracranial neoplasms. Neurology. 1985;35(2):219–26.
120. Patchell RA, Tibbs PA, Walsh JW, Dempsey RJ, Maruyama Y, Kryscio RJ, et al. A randomized trial of surgery in the treatment of single metastases to the brain. N Engl J Med. 1990;322(8):494–500.
121. Yoo H, Kim YZ, Nam BH, Shin SH, Yang HS, Lee JS, et al. Reduced local recurrence of a single brain metastasis through microscopic total resection. J Neurosurg. 2009;110(4):730–6.
122. Neves S, Mazal PR, Wanschitz J, Rudnay AC, Drlicek M, Czech T, et al. Pseudogliomatous growth pattern of anaplastic small cell carcinomas metastatic to the brain. Clin Neuropathol. 2001;20(1):38–42.
123. Baumert BG, Rutten I, Dehing-Oberije C, Twijnstra A, Dirx MJM, Debougnoux-Huppertz RMTL, et al. A pathology-based substrate for target definition in radiosurgery of brain metastases. Int J Radiat Oncol Biol Phys. 2006;66(1):187–94.
124. Berghoff AS, Rajky O, Winkler F, Bartsch R, Furtner J, Hainfellner JA, et al. Invasion patterns in brain metastases of solid cancers. Neuro Oncol. 2013;15(12):1664–72.
125. Kamp MA, Rapp M, Slotty PJ, Turowski B, Sadat H, Smuga M, et al. Incidence of local in-brain progression after supramarginal resection of cerebral metastases. Acta Neurochir. 2015;157(6):905–11.
126. Chua TH, See AAQ, Ang BT, King NKK. Awake craniotomy for resection of brain metastases: a systematic review. World Neurosurg. 2018;120:e1128–e35.
127. Brown T, Shah AH, Bregy A, Shah NH, Thambuswamy M, Barbarite E, et al. Awake craniotomy for brain tumor resection: the rule rather than the exception? J Neurosurg Anesthesiol. 2013;25(3):240–7.
128. Regine WF, Huhn JL, Patchell RA, St. Clair WH, Strottmann J, Meigooni A, et al. Risk of symptomatic brain tumor recurrence and neurologic deficit after radiosurgery alone in patients with newly diag-

onised brain metastases: results and implications. Int J Radiat Oncol Biol Phys. 2002;52(2):333–8.
129. Aoyama H, Shirato H, Tago M, Nakagawa K, Toyoda T, Hatano K, et al. Stereotactic radiosurgery plus whole-brain radiation therapy vs stereotactic radiosurgery alone for treatment of brain metastases: a randomized controlled trial. JAMA. 2006;295(21):2483–91.
130. Petrovich Brennan NM, Whalen S, de Morales BD, O'Shea JP, Norton IH, Golby AJ. Object naming is a more sensitive measure of speech localization than number counting: converging evidence from direct cortical stimulation and fMRI. Neuroimage. 2007;37:S100–S8.
131. Piccioni F, Fanzio M. Management of anesthesia in awake craniotomy. Minerva Anestesiol. 2008;74(7-8):393–408.
132. Weingarten DM, Asthagiri AR, Butman JA, Sato S, Wiggs EA, Damaska B, et al. Cortical mapping and frameless stereotactic navigation in the high-field intraoperative magnetic resonance imaging suite: technical note. J Neurosurg. 2009;111(6):1185–90.
133. Ulmer S, Braga TA, Barker FG 2nd, Lev MH, Gonzalez RG, Henson JW. Clinical and radiographic features of peritumoral infarction following resection of glioblastoma. Neurology. 2006;67(9):1668–70.
134. Smith JS, Cha S, Mayo MC, McDermott MW, Parsa AT, Chang SM, et al. Serial diffusion-weighted magnetic resonance imaging in cases of glioma: distinguishing tumor recurrence from postresection injury. J Neurosurg. 2005;103(3):428–38.
135. Berger MS, Kincaid J, Ojemann GA, Lettich E. Brain mapping techniques to maximize resection, safety, and seizure control in children with brain tumors. Neurosurgery. 1989;25(5):786–92.
136. Keles GE, Lundin DA, Lamborn KR, Chang EF, Ojemann G, Berger MS. Intraoperative subcortical stimulation mapping for hemispheric perirolandic gliomas located within or adjacent to the descending motor pathways: evaluation of morbidity and assessment of functional outcome in 294 patients. J Neurosurg. 2004;100(3):369–75.
137. Bello L, Gallucci M, Fava M, Carrabba G, Giussani C, Acerbi F, et al. Intraoperative subcortical language tract mapping guides surgical removal of gliomas involving speech areas. Neurosurgery. 2007;60(1):67–80; discussion 82.
138. Duffau H, Capelle L, Sichez N, Denvil D, Lopes M, Sichez JP, et al. Intraoperative mapping of the subcortical language pathways using direct stimulations. An anatomo-functional study. Brain. 2002;125(Pt 1):199–214.
139. Javadi SA, Nabavi A, Giordano M, Faghihzadeh E, Samii A. Evaluation of diffusion tensor imaging-based tractography of the corticospinal tract: a correlative study with intraoperative magnetic resonance imaging and direct electrical subcortical stimulation. Neurosurgery. 2017;80(2):287–99.
140. Ohue S, Kohno S, Inoue A, Yamashita D, Harada H, Kumon Y, et al. Accuracy of diffusion tensor magnetic resonance imaging-based tractography for surgery of gliomas near the pyramidal tract: a significant correlation between subcortical electrical stimulation and postoperative tractography. Neurosurgery. 2012;70(2):283–93; discussion 294
141. Ohue S, Kohno S, Inoue A, Yamashita D, Matsumoto S, Suehiro S, et al. Surgical results of tumor resection using tractography-integrated navigation-guided fence-post catheter techniques and motor-evoked potentials for preservation of motor function in patients with glioblastomas near the pyramidal tracts. Neurosurg Rev. 2015;38(2):293–306; discussion 307.
142. Schucht P, Ghareeb F, Duffau H. Surgery for low-grade glioma infiltrating the central cerebral region: location as a predictive factor for neurological deficit, epileptological outcome, and quality of life: clinical article. J Neurosurg. 2013;119(2):318–23.
143. Berger MS, Ojemann GA. Intraoperative brain mapping techniques in neuro-oncology. Stereotact Funct Neurosurg. 1992;58(1–4):153–61.
144. Pendleton C, Zaidi HA, Chaichana KL, Raza SM, Carson BS, Cohen-Gadol AA, et al. Harvey Cushing's contributions to motor mapping: 1902-1912. Cortex. 2012;48(1):7–14.
145. Penfield W, Boldrey E. Somatic motor and sensory representation in the cerebral cortex of man as studied by electrical stimulation. Brain. 1937;60(4):389–443.
146. Whitaker HA, Ojemann GA. Graded localisation of naming from electrical stimulation mapping of left cerebral cortex. Nature. 1977;270(5632):50–1.
147. Kombos T, Süss O. Neurophysiological basis of direct cortical stimulation and applied neuroanatomy of the motor cortex: a review. Neurosurg Focus. 2009;27(4):E3.
148. Taniguchi M, Cedzich C, Schramm J. Modification of cortical stimulation for motor evoked potentials under general anesthesia: technical description. Neurosurgery. 1993;32(2):219–26.
149. Bertani G, Fava E, Casaceli G, Carrabba G, Casarotti A, Papagno C, et al. Intraoperative mapping and monitoring of brain functions for the resection of low-grade gliomas: technical considerations. Neurosurg Focus. 2009;27(4):E4.
150. Plans G, Fernández-Conejero I, Rifà-Ros X, Fernández-Coello A, Rosselló A, Gabarrós A. Evaluation of the high-frequency monopolar stimulation technique for mapping and monitoring the corticospinal tract in patients with supratentorial gliomas. a proposal for intraoperative management based on neurophysiological data analysis in a series of 92 patients. Neurosurgery. 2017;81(4):585–94.
151. Raabe A, Beck J, Schucht P, Seidel K. Continuous dynamic mapping of the corticospinal tract during surgery of motor eloquent brain tumors: evaluation of a new method. J Neurosurg. 2014;120(5):1015–24.
152. Grossman R, Nossek E, Sitt R, Hayat D, Shahar T, Barzilai O, et al. Outcome of elderly patients under-

going awake-craniotomy for tumor resection. Ann Surg Oncol. 2013;20(5):1722–8.
153. Pallud J, Dezamis E. Functional and oncological outcomes following awake surgical resection using intraoperative cortico-subcortical functional mapping for supratentorial gliomas located in eloquent areas. Neurochirurgie. 2017;63(3):208–18.
154. Zemmoura I, Herbet G, Moritz-Gasser S, Duffau H. New insights into the neural network mediating reading processes provided by cortico-subcortical electrical mapping. Hum Brain Mapp. 2015;36(6):2215–30.
155. Verst SM, de Aguiar PHP, Joaquim MAS, Vieira VG, Sucena ABC, Maldaun MVC. Monopolar 250-500 Hz language mapping: results of 41 patients. Clin Neurophysiol Pract. 2019;4:1–8.
156. Krivosheya D, Rao G, Tummala S, Kumar V, Suki D, Bastos DCA, et al. Impact of multi-modality monitoring using direct electrical stimulation to determine corticospinal tract shift and integrity in tumors using the intraoperative MRI. J Neurol Surg A Cent Eur Neurosurg. 2021;82(04):375–80.
157. Shiban E, Krieg SM, Haller B, Buchmann N, Obermueller T, Boeckh-Behrens T, et al. Intraoperative subcortical motor evoked potential stimulation: how close is the corticospinal tract? J Neurosurg. 2015;123(3):711–20.
158. Kanno A, Mikuni N. Evaluation of language function under awake craniotomy. Neurol Med Chir. 2015;55(5):367–73.
159. Leal RTM, Barcellos BM, Landeiro JA. Technical aspects of awake craniotomy with mapping for brain tumors in a limited resource setting. World Neurosurg. 2018;113:67–72.
160. Mandonnet E, Winkler PA, Duffau H. Direct electrical stimulation as an input gate into brain functional networks: principles, advantages and limitations. Acta Neurochir. 2010;152(2):185–93.
161. Krieg SM, Shiban E, Droese D, Gempt J, Buchmann N, Pape H, et al. Predictive value and safety of intraoperative neurophysiological monitoring with motor evoked potentials in glioma surgery. Neurosurgery. 2012;70(5):1060–70; discussion 1070-1.
162. Ritaccio AL, Brunner P, Schalk G. Electrical stimulation mapping of the brain: basic principles and emerging alternatives. J Clin Neurophysiol. 2018;35(2):86–97.
163. Swift JR, Coon WG, Guger C, Brunner P, Bunch M, Lynch T, et al. Passive functional mapping of receptive language areas using electrocorticographic signals. Clin Neurophysiol. 2018;129(12):2517–24.
164. Gasser T, Szelenyi A, Senft C, Muragaki Y, Sandalcioglu IE, Sure U, et al. Intraoperative MRI and functional mapping. In: Pamir MN, Seifert V, Kiris T, editors. Intraoperative imaging. Vienna: Springer; 2011. p. 61–5.
165. Lu J-F, Zhang H, Wu J-S, Yao C-J, Zhuang D-X, Qiu T-M, et al. "Awake" intraoperative functional MRI (ai-fMRI) for mapping the eloquent cortex: is it possible in awake craniotomy? NeuroImage Clin. 2013;2:132–42.
166. Hirschberg H, Samset E, Hol PK, Tillung T, Lote K. Impact of intraoperative MRI on the surgical results for high-grade gliomas. Minim Invasive Neurosurg. 2005;48(02):77–84.
167. Coburger J, Merkel A, Scherer M, Schwartz F, Gessler F, Roder C, et al. Low-grade glioma surgery in intraoperative magnetic resonance imaging: results of a multicenter retrospective assessment of the German Study Group for Intraoperative Magnetic Resonance Imaging. Neurosurgery. 2016;78(6):775–86.
168. Hatiboglu MA, Weinberg JS, Suki D, Rao G, Prabhu SS, Shah K, et al. Impact of intraoperative high-field magnetic resonance imaging guidance on glioma surgery: a prospective volumetric analysis. Neurosurgery. 2009;64(6):1073–81; discussion 1081.
169. Tuominen J, Yrjänä S, Ukkonen A, Koivukangas J. Awake craniotomy may further improve neurological outcome of intraoperative MRI-guided brain tumor surgery. Acta Neurochir. 2013;155(10):1805–12.
170. Wu JS, Gong X, Song YY, Zhuang DX, Yao CJ, Qiu TM, et al. 3.0-T intraoperative magnetic resonance imaging-guided resection in cerebral glioma surgery: interim analysis of a prospective, randomized, triple-blind, parallel-controlled trial. Neurosurgery. 2014;61(Suppl 1):145–54.
171. Pichierri A, Bradley M, Iyer V. Intraoperative magnetic resonance imaging–guided glioma resections in awake or asleep settings and feasibility in the context of a public health system. World Neurosurg. 2019;3:100022.
172. Reyns N, Leroy HA, Delmaire C, Derre B, Le-Rhun E, Lejeune JP. Intraoperative MRI for the management of brain lesions adjacent to eloquent areas. Neurochirurgie. 2017;63(3):181–8.
173. Mehdorn HM, Schwartz F, Becker J, editors. Awake craniotomy for tumor resection: further optimizing therapy of brain tumors. In: Trends in reconstructive neurosurgery. Cham: Springer; 2017.
174. Motomura K, Natsume A, Iijima K, Kuramitsu S, Fujii M, Yamamoto T, et al. Surgical benefits of combined awake craniotomy and intraoperative magnetic resonance imaging for gliomas associated with eloquent areas. J Neurosurg. 2017;127(4):790–7.
175. Zhuang D-X, Wu J-S, Yao C-J, Qiu T-M, Lu J-F, Zhu F-P, et al. Intraoperative multi-information-guided resection of dominant-sided insular gliomas in a 3-T intraoperative magnetic resonance imaging integrated neurosurgical suite. World Neurosurg. 2016;89:84–92.
176. Hall WA, Liu H, Martin AJ, Pozza CH, Maxwell RE, Truwit CL. Safety, efficacy, and functionality of high-field strength interventional magnetic resonance imaging for neurosurgery. Neurosurgery. 2000;46(3):632–41; discussion 641-2.
177. Groshev A, Padalia D, Patel S, Garcia-Getting R, Sahebjam S, Forsyth PA, et al. Clinical outcomes

from maximum-safe resection of primary and metastatic brain tumors using awake craniotomy. Clin Neurol Neurosurg. 2017;157:25–30.
178. Kwinta BM, Myszka AM, Bigaj MM, Krzyżewski RM, Starowicz-Filip A. Intra- and postoperative adverse events in awake craniotomy for intrinsic supratentorial brain tumors. Neurol Sci. 2021;42(4):1437–41.
179. Southwell DG, Hervey-Jumper SL, Perry DW, Berger MS. Intraoperative mapping during repeat awake craniotomy reveals the functional plasticity of adult cortex. J Neurosurg. 2016;124(5):1460–9.
180. Eseonu CI, ReFaey K, Garcia O, John A, Quiñones-Hinojosa A, Tripathi P. Awake craniotomy anesthesia: a comparison of the monitored anesthesia care and asleep-awake-asleep techniques. World Neurosurg. 2017;104:679–86.
181. Dilmen OK, Akcil EF, Oguz A, Vehid H, Tunali Y. Comparison of conscious sedation and asleep-awake-asleep techniques for awake craniotomy. J Clin Neurosci. 2017;35:30–4.
182. Lobo FA, Wagemakers M, Absalom AR. Anaesthesia for awake craniotomy. Br J Anaesth. 2016;116(6):740–4.
183. Yuan Y, Peizhi Z, Xiang W, Yanhui L, Ruofei L, Shu J, et al. Intraoperative seizures and seizures outcome in patients undergoing awake craniotomy. J Neurosurg Sci. 2019;63(3):301–7.
184. Nossek E, Matot I, Shahar T, Barzilai O, Rapoport Y, Gonen T, et al. Intraoperative seizures during awake craniotomy: incidence and consequences: analysis of 477 patients. Neurosurgery. 2013;73(1):135–40; discussion 1340.
185. Gonen T, Grossman R, Sitt R, Nossek E, Yanaki R, Cagnano E, et al. Tumor location and IDH1 mutation may predict intraoperative seizures during awake craniotomy. J Neurosurg. 2014;121(5):1133–8.
186. Eseonu CI, Rincon-Torroella J, Lee YM, ReFaey K, Tripathi P, Quinones-Hinojosa A. Intraoperative seizures in awake craniotomy for perirolandic glioma resections that undergo cortical mapping. J Neurol Surg A Cent Eur Neurosurg. 2018;79(3):239–46.
187. Nossek E, Matot I, Shahar T, Barzilai O, Rapoport Y, Gonen T, et al. Failed awake craniotomy: a retrospective analysis in 424 patients undergoing craniotomy for brain tumor. J Neurosurg. 2013;118(2):243–9.
188. Pereira LCM, Oliveira KM, L'Abbate GL, Sugai R, Ferreira JA, da Motta LA. Outcome of fully awake craniotomy for lesions near the eloquent cortex: analysis of a prospective surgical series of 79 supratentorial primary brain tumors with long follow-up. Acta Neurochir. 2008;151(10):1215–30.
189. Zhang JJY, Lee KS, Voisin MR, Hervey-Jumper SL, Berger MS, Zadeh G. Awake craniotomy for resection of supratentorial glioblastoma: a systematic review and meta-analysis. Neurooncol Adv. 2020;2(1):vdaa111.
190. Bello L, Fava E, Casaceli G, Bertani G, Carrabba G, Papagno C, et al. Intraoperative mapping for tumor resection. Neuroimaging Clin. 2009;19(4):597–614.
191. Saito T, Muragaki Y, Tamura M, Maruyama T, Nitta M, Tsuzuki S, et al. Awake craniotomy with transcortical motor evoked potential monitoring for resection of gliomas in the precentral gyrus: utility for predicting motor function. J Neurosurg. 2019;132(4):987–97.
192. Khan F, Amatya B, Drummond K, Galea M. Effectiveness of integrated multidisciplinary rehabilitation in primary brain cancer survivors in an Australian community cohort: a controlled clinical trial. J Rehabil Med. 2014;46(8):754–60.
193. Goettel N, Bharadwaj S, Venkatraghavan L, Mehta J, Bernstein M, Manninen PH. Dexmedetomidine vs propofol-remifentanil conscious sedation for awake craniotomy: a prospective randomized controlled trial. Br J Anaesth. 2016;116(6):811–21.
194. Southwell DG, Birk HS, Han SJ, Li J, Sall JW, Berger MS. Resection of gliomas deemed inoperable by neurosurgeons based on preoperative imaging studies. J Neurosurg. 2018;129(3):567–75.
195. Suarez-Meade P, Marenco-Hillembrand L, Prevatt C, Murguia-Fuentes R, Mohamed A, Alsaeed T, et al. Awake vs. asleep motor mapping for glioma resection: a systematic review and meta-analysis. Acta Neurochir. 2020;162(7):1709–20.
196. Lu VM, Phan K, Rovin RA. Comparison of operative outcomes of eloquent glioma resection performed under awake versus general anesthesia: a systematic review and meta-analysis. Clin Neurol Neurosurg. 2018;169:121–7.
197. Bu LH, Zhang J, Lu JF, Wu JS. Glioma surgery with awake language mapping versus generalized anesthesia: a systematic review. Neurosurg Rev. 2021;44(4):1997–2011.
198. Duffau H, Lopes M, Arthuis F, Bitar A, Sichez J-P, Van Effenterre R, et al. Contribution of intraoperative electrical stimulations in surgery of low grade gliomas: a comparative study between two series without (1985–96) and with (1996–2003) functional mapping in the same institution. J Neurol Neurosurg Psychiatry. 2005;76(6):845–51.
199. Gravesteijn BY, Keizer ME, Vincent AJPE, Schouten JW, Stolker RJ, Klimek M. Awake craniotomy versus craniotomy under general anesthesia for the surgical treatment of insular glioma: choices and outcomes. Neurol Res. 2018;40(2):87–96.
200. Martino J, Gomez E, Bilbao JL, Dueñas JC, Vázquez-Barquero A. Cost-utility of maximal safe resection of WHO grade II gliomas within eloquent areas. Acta Neurochir. 2013;155(1):41–50.
201. Gerritsen JKW, Viëtor CL, Rizopoulos D, Schouten JW, Klimek M, Dirven CMF, et al. Awake craniotomy versus craniotomy under general anesthesia without surgery adjuncts for supratentorial glioblastoma in eloquent areas: a retrospective matched case-control study. Acta Neurochir. 2019;161(2):307–15.

Awake Craniotomy in Epilepsy Surgery <Awake Craniotomy, Epilepsy, Mapping>

Amirhossein Larijani and Ahmad Pour-Rashidi

1 Introduction

Maximal safe resection of gliomas and preserving eloquent areas is the aim of surgery. In epilepsy surgery, the goal is resection of the epileptogenic zone to control epilepsy while preserving function. To identify the epileptogenic zone electrophysiological and neuroradiological studies should be done. Non-invasive studies, such as magnetic resonance imaging (MRI) and magnetoencephalography (MEG) have progressed markedly [1, 2]; whereas, identification of epileptogenic zones requires invasive evaluation. Epileptogenic foci such as focal cortical dysplasia (FCD) type 1 often show minimal histopathological and imaging changes. These foci are often located in eloquent areas requiring awake surgery.

Functional mapping can also be performed in awake surgery, allowing identification of eloquent areas and these functions can be continuously monitored during lesionectomy. Second, intraoperative electrocorticography (ECoG) can be recorded without being influenced by anesthesia. Therefore, awake surgery provides almost as much ECoG information in the interictal phase as those of step-2 chronic invasive ECoG recording in the patients' ward, which is usually problematic, and considered an important cause of epilepsy patient drop-out from presurgical evaluation [3].

Resective surgery for epilepsy is often divided into temporal and extra-temporal epilepsy surgery and is considered a well-established treatment [4]. Every case is processed through a team-based work-up of possible risks vs. potential benefits of the prospective resection [4]. Awake craniotomy has been used in epilepsy surgery during the twentieth century by such prominent neurosurgeons as Foerster, Penfield, and Ojemann. Publications by Penfield greatly contributed to the early understanding of function localization [5–8], although the present view of brain function has developed into a deeper understanding of functions as networks instead of localizations (referred to as hodotopy), or connectomics rather than topography. This philosophy of brain function has had broad implications in intraoperative mapping in surgery for low-grade gliomas [9, 10]. During surgery, direct cor-

A. Larijani (✉)
Department of Neurosurgery, Shahid Madani Hospital, Alborz University of Medical Sciences, Alborz, Iran

A. Pour-Rashidi
Department of Neurosurgery, Tehran University of Medical Sciences, Tehran, Iran
e-mail: apourrashidi@sina.tums.ac.ir

A. Pour-Rashidi, J. Aarabi (eds.), *The Principles of Successful Awake Craniotomy*, https://doi.org/10.1007/978-981-99-2985-6_3

tical and subcortical stimulation with a handheld probe is regarded as the gold standard to map eloquent areas in the cortex and important tracts. The accuracy is greater than with the non-invasive methods mentioned above. Awake surgery may sometimes allow a larger resection, but whether this leads to better seizure outcome has not been thoroughly studied.

In the twenty-first century, several articles about epilepsy surgery performed on awake patients have been published [11, 12]. Several studies concerning understanding memory function have been published based on patients undergoing awake surgery for epilepsy [13]. Most studies on awake surgery in epilepsy have, however, included tumor patients. Few studies have been published [14–16] with a technical description of awake surgery of epileptogenic lesions in eloquent areas.

Cortical neuroplasticity is the ability of cortical organization rearrangement, through a dynamic continuous process allowing remodeling of the cortical neuronal synaptic organization, to retain brain functions which is sustained by "brain connectome" [17]. In glioma surgery, the knowledge of cortical neuroplasticity and connectomics is important to achieve a maximal safe resection. Intraoperative cortical and subcortical mapping during awake surgery is now the gold standard for attaining these results. Connectomics, in epilepsy surgery, is largely considered for the description of the organization of the abnormal epileptic networks [18]. Nevertheless, this approach for functional mapping is not as developed as it is in glioma surgery.

In this chapter, the role of awake surgery for epilepsy is described based on the techniques developed for tumor removal, which should be improved to focus on epileptic networks in addition to functional mapping. The importance of cortical neuroplasticity and connectomics is emphasized and a review concerning the development of adjunct intraoperative mapping techniques for better epileptogenic zone resection is presented. At the end of this chapter, current clinical outcomes and implications of AC in resective epilepsy surgery are discussed.

2 Indications and Patient Selection

The first awake craniotomies were initially performed on patients with drug-resistant epilepsy with the aim of functional cortical mapping and electrocorticography [19, 20]. In contrast, intraoperative stimulations for mapping led to some misunderstandings related to partial seizure attacks. Interictal electrocorticography appeared to have a limited impact on the definition of the ictal-onset zone, and the comprehension of the seizure as a dynamic process by Jean Talairach [21] led to promote invasive presurgical investigation based on long-term intracranial ictal recordings.

The first guidelines about surgery in drug-resistant epilepsy were published in 2003 by the American Academy of Neurology and updated in 2006 by the International League Against Epilepsy [22]. Randomized trials, such as the Early Randomized Surgical Epilepsy Trial, are few, but reflect interest concerning early surgery in terms of quality-of-life improvement and seizure control [23]. Retrospective studies led to similar conclusions and suggested that short duration of epilepsy and young age were important factors of seizure control, both in temporal and extratemporal epilepsy [24–26]. Epilepsy generates poor cortical neuroplasticity. Moreover, focal epilepsy is considered a long-term disease like low-grade glioma and neuroplasticity does not seem to operate in the same way. In comparison with low-grade glioma where functions can be redistributed among larger networks, in focal epilepsy, functions of cortical areas are usually close to what is described in "localizationist" atlases and cannot be redistributed.

In contrast with low-grade gliomas, epilepsy is a cortical pathology and resection is not intended to involve the white matter tracts. Cortical resection in the eloquent area, such as ictal-onset zone, will result in an expected neurologic impairment which will recover within weeks or months if the connectome is preserved, as seen after low-grade glioma surgery [27]. Before adopting such an approach for a functional neurosurgery, the probability of recovery should be determined through prelesional investigation that has been similarly described by neuro-oncology [28].

In patients with epilepsy, another type of neuroplasticity should be considered whereupon the white matter pathologic plasticity modifies the anatomy and that epileptic networks are sustained by pathologic aberrant pathways that are not supposed to sustain any function with no role in connectome. These pathologic structures are described at a local level [29] as well as on long-distance trajectories [30–33], and are constituted of abnormal fiber tracts, distinct from the normal white matter anatomy. For instance, fiber projections from periventricular heterotopias to distant neocortical areas are obviously sustained by non-anatomic pathways even if they may cross them [34]. Moreover, patterns of increased connectivity related to the epileptogenic zone, coupled with decreased connectivity in widespread distal networks have been found, and are correlated to the severity and the duration of the disease [35]. Those pathologic networks may provide a benefit in terms of seizure-spreading limitation but may also impair physiologic networks of the connectome and have a negative impact on function. This could lead to defining new therapeutic strategies for patients in whom the ictal-onset zone cannot be respected.

In some patients, investigations report an expansion of large cortical areas in epileptic networks, even in distant regions. These patients are usually not eligible for surgery because of risk of injury to the connectome and following permanent neurologic impairment. In these cases, small stereotactic lesions in the epileptic network could improve the epilepsy [36]. Awake mapping could identify the connectome and the crucial pathways within the white matter as well as locate the white matter tracks involved in the seizure spreading. By summation of these two networks, it would be possible to define targets which destruct the epileptic network without impairing the connectome. Epilepsy surgeries have tried to overcome the issue of primary cortical areas [37] but approaches to these crucial eloquent locations may impose severe neurologic deficits because these cortical areas are usually the only input or output of essential white matter pathways. Injury to these areas may relate to a permanent and complete disconnection of a part of the connectome with no recovery through neuroplasticity. Functional mapping of the involved area may help to define the essential subcortical connections of the connectome and, in defining the connections, they could be disconnected without desynchronizing the connectome. This would be a palliative approach for decreasing the severity of the seizures by altering the epileptic network [38].

3 Technical Nuances

There are three different approaches of performing awake craniotomy: asleep–awake–asleep (SAS) developed and modified by W. Penfield, K. Hall, and D. Ingvar in the 1950s; awake–awake–awake (AAA), suggested by E. Hansen in 2013; and monitored anesthesia care (MAC) [39–43]. These methods have their disadvantages and advantages and have been widely reported in literature [41, 42, 44]. "MAC" is associated with lower awake craniotomy failure rate, shorter procedure time, a trend toward reduced length of hospitalization, and incidence of nausea and vomiting compared with "SAS". There is a higher rate of intraoperative seizures during "MAC" [44]. In "AAA" method, major side effects of general anesthesia or sedation are reduced or even avoided. These side effects and complications of anesthetics have actually been described for awake craniotomy using "SAS" [39].

Preoperative evaluations, including 1.5 T and 3 T MRI, fMRI, diffusion tensor imaging tractography, and long-term electroencephalogram video monitoring to identify the source of pathological activity, have an important role in surgical planning.

Prior to the surgery, the patients are informed about the surgical intervention plan, the possible risks and complications of the surgery, and the alleged uncomfortable sensations associated with craniotomy. The sound phenomena related to surgical intervention (sound of electrocoagulation, perforator, vacuum aspirator, and pneumatic drill) and possible inconveniences (i.e., forced position on the operating table, the probability of aphasia occurrence, or uncontrolled muscle contractions during cortical stimulation, seizure development) are described to the patients.

As described in previous study of Sitnikov et al. [39], fixation of the patients' head on the operating table is performed under local anesthesia with 5 mL of 0.75% Ropivacaine (Naropin) mixed with 5 mL of 1% lidocaine, which is administered in equal amounts in the region of the three-point Mayfield clamp fixation. The heating system is used for patients intraoperatively to maintain a comfortable body temperature in the range of 36–37 °C and to prevent a thermoregulatory tremor. The size of the planned trepanation exceeds the area of the pathological focus determined by neuronavigation between 2 and 4 cm to perform cortical function mapping and corticography.

Planned skin incision line is infiltrated with a mixture of 0.75% ropivacaine (Naropin) and 1% lidocaine in a 1:1 ratio. If it is necessary to dissect the temporal muscle, it is infiltrated with the same solution. After local anesthesia is achieved, a skin incision and the subsequent surgery stages are performed.

When trepanation and dura mater are incised, all patients undergo corticography with strip electrodes and grid electrodes. The brain is covered with electrodes and by using the neuronavigation system, it is possible to focus on pathological areas as well as adjacent cortical regions at a distance of not less than 1.5–2 cm from the margins of the lesion.

The choice of tests for cortical function mapping is determined by the anatomic location of the lesion. Patients undergo bipolar biphasic stimulation with rectangular current using the cortical stimulator with parameters 1 ms/phase, 60 Hz, and 2–20 mA for motor function mapping. Motor response is registered on the contralateral side with subcutaneous needle electrodes placed on mm. orbicularis oris, orbicularis oculi, masseter, trapezius, deltoid, triceps, brachioradialis, abductor policies brevis, abductor digitis minimi, quadriceps, anterior tibialis, and abductor halluces.

To identify speech centers, object naming tests and reading tests along with a direct monopolar monophasic electrical stimulation with a stepwise current intensity increase from 2 to 11 mA under control of the intraoperative corticography are used prior to the occurrence of verbal disturbances or after discharges on electrocorticography. Evaluation of seizure control in the postoperative period is carried out according to Engel's scale and ILAE scale.

4 Intraoperative Adjuncts

4.1 SEEG Recordings and Electrical Mapping

The choice of deep stereoelectroencephalography (SEEG) monitoring is based on three principles: [45] the cortico-subcortical location of the FCD between the superior temporal sulcus and the inferior insular sulcus; [46] the need to explore mesial temporal structures as up to 43% of temporal lobe FCD that may be associated with hippocampal sclerosis [47] in 'dual pathology'; and finally [48], the functional boundaries of the FCD especially at the subcortical level; because, the inferior fronto-occipital fasciculus ran at its mesial and superior borders. This pathway is known to be implicated in semantic word processing [49].

4.2 Intraoperative Stimulation Mapping Considerations

The use of intraoperative direct cortical stimulation for epilepsy surgery in cases of FCD is not new [50–53]. It has always been used with the purpose of optimizing the quality of resection while preserving function. A few studies compared positive simulation with invasive monitoring to intraoperative stimulation. In contrast, when functional tissue was detected by preoperative stimulation, it was not resected and other techniques such as multiple subpial transections were performed with unsatisfactory results [54]. This supports the series of Chassoux et al. [55], where 29 patients with FCD explored with SEEG,

5 had partial resection of the EZ for functional reasons and all of them resulted in a negative outcome (Engel III and IV). Nevertheless, in some selected cases functional cortex overlapping with FCD has been removed, such as in the motor cortex of the face, which could be compensated due to its bilateral representation [56].

Awake mapping made it possible to identify the crucial cortical sites before resection to preserve them and to pursue removal until the stimulation-induced reproducible language disturbances within the white matter. This concept of surgery according to functional boundaries has been widely used in tumor surgery, especially for slow-growing lesions such as low-grade gliomas [57–63].

4.3 Discrepancies Between SEEG and Intraoperative Stimulation

Two major factors may explain these discrepancies. First, the stimulation intensity may offer some clarity. Language disturbances were obtained at 10 mA in the SEEG explorations, while in awake direct electrostimulation, the current intensity was 2.5 mA (i.e., as the mean reported threshold by several authors [55, 58, 62], which is between 2 and 6 mA). This means that, due to the high-intensity current used through SEEG leads (never reached when using direct cortico-subcortical stimulation in the awake patient), even in the absence of after-discharge patterns or of induced seizure during SEEG stimulation, there is no evidence that the impairment was not due to a blocking of more distant areas. Second, intraoperatively, once the threshold of the language had been set, if stimulation induced a reproducible impairment, the surgeon could be certain that this area was essential for function [62], both at cortical and subcortical levels [49]. Conversely, the lack of reproducibility of language disturbances during repeated SEEG stimulation seemed to indicate that the participation of the areas mapped was not essential or could be compensated. This plasticity phenomenon may be a new concept in epilepsy surgery but not in oncological brain mapping surgery. In fact, the degree of plasticity seems to be related to the growing curve of the lesion. In cases of slow-growing lesions such as low-grade gliomas (4 mm/year on average) [64], the progressive invasion of functional areas induces a reshaping which explains, in part, the fact that almost all these patients had no neurological deficits [65]. This kind of compensation has been described during glioma surgery of sensorimotor regions, language sites (e.g., Broca's area) as well as associative areas such as the insula and the claustrum [55, 66]. Moreover, years of seizures arising from a focus in a highly functional area may mimic a chronic lesion and induce plasticity with reshaping of functional areas and has been mentioned by Burneo et al., [67]. In this MEG study, patients with FCD in eloquent regions (rolandic and calcarin cortex) showed a reshaping of functional areas around the FCD before any surgery. This brain plasticity can be very useful for the neurosurgeon since it may make it possible to perform a complete removal of the FCD and the EZ without permanent worsening of speech.

There are some studies about memory mapping in patients with subdural and deep electrodes implantation [68–70]. In the study conducted by Coleshill et al. [68], left hippocampal stimulation was related to word-recognition memory deficits, while right hippocampal stimulation was related to face-recognition memory deficits [68]. Tani et al., [70] demonstrated that electrical stimulation at the parahippocampus could predict functional outcomes for memory [70]. According to these reports, functional mapping of memory function may be possible, but it is limited by the short time in an intraoperative setting.

Working memory is another high cognitive function field of interest for intraoperative mapping [71, 72]. A case report in 2007 presented a patient with an epileptogenic lesion in the left dorsolateral prefrontal cortex where working memory mapping was performed during in-ward chronic ECoG recording [71]. The surgery revealed positive areas for some tasks for working memory, such as an *n*-back task. However, because those areas were considered the epileptogenic zone, they were resected. Postoperatively, the patient demonstrated deterioration of working memory. It was concluded that working memory mapping correlated with surgical outcomes, and it was justified. Matsui et al. [72] reported that intraoperative dorsolateral prefrontal cortex (DLPFC) stimulation caused positive responses in some attention tasks, such as the color Stroop test, which may be related to working memory [72].

It remains challenging to perform intraoperative mapping for higher cognition. There is a need for improvement of tasks that can be performed during the short intraoperative period with high sensitivity and specificity, as well as reproducibility and safety. Furthermore, even if a higher cognitive area is identified whether it should be resected or retained remains an issue, which depends on whether higher cognitive function or seizure control is the priority.

5 Complications and Morbidities

Awake craniotomy complications including anesthesia and surgery are related. The first one includes upper respiratory tract obstruction (hypoxia, conversion to general anesthesia, hypertension/hypotension), tachycardia/bradycardia, nausea (vomiting), and toxic effects of local anesthetic (pain, poor patient cooperation, and agitation). The surgical complications can be presented with focal seizures, generalized seizures, the appearance of a neurological deficit (aphasia, paresis), bleeding, cerebral edema, and air embolism [73, 74].

According to the meta-analysis of literature published between 2007 and 2015, which included the results of 5945 awake craniotomies in 5931 patients, in the group of patients who underwent craniotomy under the sleep-awake-sleep protocol, the most common complications were distributed as follows: intraoperative seizures 8%, new neurological deficit 17%, and the conversion to general anesthesia 2% [30]. The index of the impossibility to proceed further with awake craniotomy (awake craniotomy failure) was assessed independently including laryngeal mask leak, respiratory failure, intraoperative bleeding, intraoperative anxiety and pain, cerebral edema, convulsive seizures, and air embolism, were 2% and practically independent of the method used [75–81].

Nossek et al. [82] analyzed 477 interventions in their study under "MAC" protocol (remifentanil + propofol in low doses in the beginning and in the end of surgical intervention with the absence of medication during the awake phase); the incidence of intraoperative seizures reached 12.6%, while in 37 patients surgical intervention became impossible due to complications and in 7 patients the development of seizures led to converting to general anesthesia [82].

Drugs frequently used for awake craniotomy are propofol, remifentanil, dexmedetomidine, and their combinations [80–82]. Recently, a greater preference has been given to dexmedetomidine, a highly selective alfa-2-receptor agonist, the sedative effect of which is exerted by reducing the excitation of locus coeruleus noradrenergic neurons (locus coeruleus-basic noradrenergic nucleus located under tegmentum, in the posterior area of the rostral pons in the lateral floor of the fourth ventricle) [83].

The main advantage of dexmedetomidine is the ability to keep the epileptic activity unchanged which enables its use while performing intraoperative corticography in cases of epilepsy and epileptogenic lesions [84]. However, there are reports that an increase in drug concentration in plasma reduces the amplitude of the induced motor potentials and may lead to incorrect interpretation of the results of neurophysiological monitoring of motor responses [85].

In contrast to the previous statements about the harmlessness of dexmedetomidine in neurosurgical anesthetics, the US Department of Health and Human Services (USDHHS) and the Office of Food and Drug Administration (FDA) reports which were published in 2016 contain 37 reports of the various side effects caused by the use of this drug, particularly in pediatric practice. Severe hypotension and bradycardia, prolonged QT syndrome, fulminant hepatitis, acute adrenal insufficiency, and encephalopathy are listed among the complications [86].

The use of locoregional anesthesia and local scalp anesthesia at the incision site has also been widely discussed in literature. Mostly, the authors [87, 88] used a combination of locoregional anesthesia with local anesthesia of the scalp incision area using various combinations of local anesthetics. Their meta-analysis confirmed the efficacy of anesthesia of the nerve branches innervating the scalp, including the achievement of postoperative analgesia [89]. However, it should be noted that even with adequate technique, locoregional anesthesia carries the potential risk of complications such as toxic local anesthetic effect, systemic hypertension, hematoma formation, and peripheral nerve damage [87, 88]. Certainly, the routine use of locoregional anesthesia in combination with general anesthesia under the "SAS" protocol multiplies the risks of surgical intervention frequently. The possibility of the emergence of uncontrolled adverse reactions during the administration of sedatives or local anesthetics leads to the use of exotic methods such as electroacupuncture in neurosurgical practice [90].

6 Efficacy and Outcome

Complete resection of MRI-demarcated and ECoG abnormal lesions are the best predictive factors for seizure control results [91, 92]. Studies have yielded conflicting results in terms of the correlation between the extent of resection in the irritative zone, observed by intraoperative ECoG, and epilepsy outcomes after supratotal resection, which included a further 5–10 mm margin increase of normal tissue. The seizure freedom rate is approximately 86–92% versus 8–77% after incomplete resection [93–95]. However, recent studies have suggested that there is no correlation between resection of the irritative zone identified in ECoG and epilepsy outcome [95, 96]. There is no agreement about whether residual spikes in the post-resection ECoG predict seizure outcome [97]. To interpret post-resection ECoG, in addition to the residual spikes from residual epileptogenesis, newly developed spikes should be considered, including a spike burst–suppression pattern caused by cortical isolation [98], surgical injury of the cortex [99], and activation of a secondary focus by partial resection of the major focus [99].

There is no relationship between all residual spikes and epileptogenesis; however, it is necessary to distinguish between epileptogenesis-related spikes and unrelated spikes [100]. High-frequency oscillation in intraoperative ECoG has recently attracted much attention as a specific biomarker of epileptogenesis and may contribute to the resolution of this issue [101–104]. Compared to general anesthesia, awake surgery does not require much consideration of the influence of anesthesia agents on ECoG recordings. Anesthesia agents used during ECoG recording may affect its findings. In children, the frequency of spikes decreases markedly in intraoperative ECoG under general anesthesia as compared to extraoperative ECoG [105]. In summary, ECoG findings are influenced by anesthesia conditions. ECoG recordings during awake surgery may provide more accurate and reliable information, although no such comparative study has been reported to date.

Recent studies reveal that the use of an awake craniotomy procedure can be valuable for complex cases of epilepsy surgery, as it allows some non-operable patients to become eligible for resective surgery with minimal risks of functional complications and acceptable post-operative improvement regarding seizure status.

The incidence of stimulation-induced seizures during awake craniotomy for gliomas reported in the literature ranges from 2.2% to 21.5% [106, 107]. There is no difference in the risk of intraoperative seizures between surgery for gliomas and epileptic lesions under awake conditions.

Functional MRI (fMRI) is performed in most centers when there is suspicion of overlap between the EZ and language cortex, which provides preliminary insight into language cortex lateralization and localization. fMRI has several advantages: it is non-invasive; requires no injection of medication; and carries virtually no risk of complication. However, there remain strong limitations to fMRI scanning in defining atypical and/or essential language areas. First, the level of spatial resolution of fMRI data is lower compared to that of typical T1-weighted anatomical MRI (the BOLD signal itself is not yet entirely understood); and second, the relationship between positive and negative BOLD signals and alterations in neural activity have not been fully elucidated [108]. Regions activated during fMRI are more extensive than those elicited by direct cortical stimulation, which could lead to a more conservative approach [109]. In contrast, SEEG stimulation provides a very focal sampling of the brain, which makes it a less sensitive technique than intraoperative cortical stimulation [110]. Therefore, intraoperative cortical stimulation is irreplaceable for functional mapping. SEEG stimulation mapping is known as a complementary method to initially assess the connectome prior to surgery which may help focus on the most relevant elements preoperatively [111].

Direct electrical stimulation in awake craniotomy is the gold standard for functional mapping due to functional pre-operative mapping. Nevertheless, there are a limited number of functions that could be tested due to the time limitation of stimulation during awake surgery. Moreover, the effect of direct electrical stimulation of a deep white matter fasciculus produces similar effects implying that the cortical area facing it has previously been removed. Multiple cortical and/or subcortical site stimulations could produce effects that do not appear when these sites are isolated, which is related to existence of interconnection on the partial overlap of subnetworks of the connectome and could be relevant for both glioma and epilepsy surgery. Ultimately, perioperative direct electrical stimulation provides invaluable information about the direct effect of a lesion.

SEEG could help to focus on the most eloquent area perioperatively. Recently, ECoG, has become a complementary instrument to improve detection of the effect of direct electric stimulation during functional mapping in glioma surgery [82].

7 Conclusion

Seizure control may be achieved by the maximal lesionectomy in awake surgery. Maximal resection of the epileptogenic zone is an important factor for seizure freedom. Awake surgery may help to improve seizure outcomes through maximal lesionectomy while preserving dominant functions by means of intraoperative ECoG and mapping information. Also, SEEG stimulation mapping is known as a complementary method to initially assess the connectome prior to surgery which may help focus on the most relevant elements preoperatively.

References

1. Englot DJ, Konrad PE, Morgan VL. Regional and global connectivity disturbances in focal epilepsy, related neurocognitive sequelae, and potential mechanistic underpinnings. Epilepsia. 2016;57:1546–57.
2. Maesawa S, Bagarinao E, Fujii M, Futamura M, Wakabayashi T. Use of network analysis to establish neurosurgical parameters in gliomas and epilepsy. Neurol Med Chir (Tokyo). 2016;56:158–69.
3. Berg AT, Vickrey BG, Langfitt JT, et al. Multicenter Study of Epilepsy Surgery: the multicenter study of epilepsy surgery: recruitment and selection for surgery. Epilepsia. 2003;44:1425–33.
4. Penfield W. Conditioning the uncommitted cortex for language learning. Brain. 1965;88(4):787–98.
5. Penfield W, Welch K. Instability of motor points and sensory points in the humancerebral cortex. Fed Proc. 1948;7(1 Pt):91.
6. Rasmussen T, Penfield W. Further studies of the sensory and motor cerebral cortex of man. Fed Proc. 1947;6(2):452–60.
7. Duffau H, et al. Contribution of intraoperative electrical stimulations in surgery of low-grade gliomas: a comparative study between two series without (1985-96) and with (1996-2003) functional mapping in the same institution. J Neurol Neurosurg Psychiatry. 2005;76(6):845–51.
8. Gras-Combe G, et al. Intraoperative subcortical electrical mapping of optic radiations in awake surgery for glioma involving visual pathways. J Neurosurg. 2012;117(3):466–73.
9. Johnson LA, et al. Direct electrical stimulation of the somatosensory cortex in humans using electrocorticography electrodes: a qualitative and quantitative report. J Neural Eng. 2013;10(3):036021.
10. Poliachik SL, et al. Tissue localization during resective epilepsy surgery. Neurosurg Focus. 2013;34(6):E8.

11. Ojemann GA, Ojemann J, Ramsey NF. Relation between functional magnetic resonance imaging (fMRI) and single neuron, local field potential (LFP) and electrocorticography (ECoG) activity in human cortex. Front Hum Neurosci. 2013;7:34.
12. Maesawa S, et al. Application of awake surgery for epilepsy in clinical practice. Neurol Med Chir (Tokyo). 2018;58(10):442–52.
13. Ojemann GA, Schoenfield-McNeill J, Corina D. The roles of human lateral temporal cortical neuronal activity in recent verbal memory encoding. Cereb Cortex. 2009;19(1):197–205.
14. Natalini D, et al. Comparison of the asleep-awake-asleep technique and monitored anesthesia care during awake craniotomy: a systematic review and meta-analysis. J Neurosurg Anesthesiol. 2020;34:e1.
15. Martinoni M, et al. Ultrasound assisted awake epilepsy surgery for type IIB focal cortical dysplasia in eloquent areas. J Neurosurg Sci. 2017;65:75.
16. Joswig H, et al. Awake perimetry testing for occipital epilepsy surgery. J Neurosurg. 2017;129:1195.
17. Kim YH, et al. Resection frequency map after awake resective surgery for nonlesional neocortical epilepsy involving eloquent areas. Acta Neurochir. 2011;153(9):1739–49.
18. Duffau H. Brain plasticity: from pathophysiological mechanisms to therapeutic applications. J Clin Neurosci. 2006;13:885–97.
19. Penfield W. Epilepsy and cerebral localization. A study of the mechanism, treatment and prevention of epilepoic seizures. Arch Neurol Psychiatr. 1942;47:875.
20. Penfield W, Jasper H. Epilepsy and the functional anatomy of the human brain. Boston: Little, Brown; 1954.
21. Talairach J, Bancaud J, Bonis A, et al. Functional stereotaxic exploration of epilepsy. Confin Neurol. 1962;22:328–31.
22. Kwan P, Arzimanoglou A, Berg AT, et al. Definition of drug resistant epilepsy: consensus proposal by the ad hoc Task Force of the ILAE Commission on Therapeutic Strategies. Epilepsia. 2010;51:1069–77.
23. Ryvlin P, Cross JH, Rheims S. Epilepsy surgery in children and adults. Lancet Neurol. 2014;13:1114–26.
24. Engel J Jr, McDermott MP, Wiebe S, et al. Early surgical therapy for drug-resistant temporal lobe epilepsy: a randomized trial. JAMA. 2012;307:922–30.
25. Langfitt JT, Wiebe S. Early surgical treatment for epilepsy. Curr Opin Neurol. 2008;21:179–83.
26. Broca P. Perte de la parole, ramollissement chronique et destruction partielle du lobe anterieur gauche. Bull Soc Anthropol. 1861;2:235–8.
27. Gil Robles S, Gelisse P, Vergani F, et al. Discrepancies between preoperative stereoencephalography language stimulation mapping and intraoperative awake mapping during resection of focal cortical dysplasia in eloquent areas. Stereotact Funct Neurosurg. 2008;86:382–90.
28. Tate MC, Herbet G, Moritz-Gasser S, et al. Probabilistic map of critical functional regions of the human cerebral cortex: Broca's area revisited. Brain. 2014;137:2773–82.
29. Cano-Lopez I, Vazquez JF, Campos A, et al. Age at surgery as a predictor of cognitive improvements in patients with drug-resistant temporal epilepsy. Epilepsy Behav. 2017;70:10–7.
30. Modo M, Hitchens TK, Liu JR, et al. Detection of aberrant hippocampal mossy fiber connections: ex vivo mesoscale diffusion MRI and microtractography with histological validation in a patient with uncontrolled temporal lobe epilepsy. Hum Brain Mapp. 2016;37:780–95.
31. Imamura H, Matsumoto R, Takaya S, et al. Network specific change in white matter integrity in mesial temporal lobe epilepsy. Epilepsy Res. 2016;120:65–72.
32. Nazem-Zadeh M-R, Bowyer SM, Moran JE, et al. MEG coherence and DTI connectivity in mTLE. Brain Topogr. 2016;29:598–622.
33. Whelan CD, Alhusaini S, O'Hanlon E, et al. White matter alterations in patients with MRI- negative temporal lobe epilepsy and their asymptomatic siblings. Epilepsia. 2015;56:1551–61.
34. Taylor PN, Han CE, Schoene-Bake J-C, et al. Structural connectivity changes in temporal lobe epilepsy: spatial features contribute more than topological measures. Neuroimage Clin. 2015;8:322–8.
35. Farquharson S, Tournier J-D, Calamante F, et al. Periventricular nodular heterotopia: detection of abnormal microanatomic fiber structures with whole-brain diffusion MR imaging tractography. Radiology. 2016;281:896–906.
36. Bourdillon P, Isnard J, Catenoix H, et al. Stereo electroencephalography- guided radiofrequency thermocoagulation (SEEG-guided RF-TC) in drug-resistant focal epilepsy: results from a 10-year experience. Epilepsia. 2017;58:85–93.
37. Devaux B, Chassoux F, Landre E, et al. Surgical resections in functional areas: report of 89 cases. Neurochirurgie. 2008;54:409–17.
38. Bourdillon P, Apra C, Guénot M, Duffau H. Similarities and differences in neuroplasticity mechanisms between brain gliomas and nonlesional epilepsy. Epilepsia. 2017;58(12):2038–47.
39. Sitnikov AR, Grigoryan YA, Mishnyakova LP. Awake craniotomy without sedation in treatment of patients with lesional epilepsy. Surg Neurol Int. 2018;9:177.
40. Hall K, Baldwin M, Norris F Jr. Succinylcholine drip during craniotomy. Anesthesiology. 1959;20:65–70.
41. Hansen E, Seemann M, Zech N, Doenitz C, Luerding R, Brawanski A, et al. Awake craniotomies without any sedation: the awake-awake-awake technique. Acta Neurochir. 2013;155:1417–24.
42. Ingvar DH, Jeppsson ST, Nordstrom L. A new form of anaesthesia in surgical treatment of focal epilepsy. Acta Anaesthesiol Scand. 1959;3:111–21.

43. Penfield W. Combined regional and general anesthesia for craniotomy and cortical exploration. Anesth Analg. 1954;33:145–55.
44. Natalini D, Ganau M, Rosenkranz R, Petrinic T, Fitzgibbon K, Antonelli M, Prisco L. Comparison of the asleep-awake-asleep technique and monitored anesthesia care during awake craniotomy: a systematic review and meta-analysis. J Neurosurg Anesthesiol. 2022;34(1):e1–e13.
45. Taylor DC, Falconer MA, Bruton CJ, Corsellis JAN. Focal dysplasia of the cerebral cortex in epilepsy. J Neurol Neurosurg Psychiatry. 1971;34:369–87.
46. Palmini A, Andermann F, Olivier A, Tampieri D, Robitaille Y. Focal neuronal migration disorders and intractable partial epilepsy: results of surgical treatment. Ann Neurol. 1991;30:750–7.
47. Fauser S, Schulze-Bonhage A, Honegger J, Carmona H, Huppertz HJ, Pantazis G, et al. Focal cortical dysplasias: surgical outcome in 67 patients in relation to histological subtypes and dual pathology. Brain. 2004;127:2406–18.
48. Semah F, Picot MC, Adam C, Broglin D, Arzimanoglou A, Bazin B, et al. Is the underlying cause of epilepsy a major prognostic factor for recurrence? Neurology. 1998;51:1256–62.
49. Duffau H, Gatignol P, Mandonnet E, Peruzzi P, Tzourio-Mazoyer N, Capelle L. New insights into the anatomo-functional connectivity of the semantic system: a study using cortico-subcortical electrostimulations. Brain. 2005;128:797–810.
50. Cohen-Gadol AA, Britton JW, Collignon FP, Bates LM, Cascino GD, Meyer FB. Nonlesional central lobule seizures: use of awake cortical mapping and subdural grid monitoring for resection of seizure focus. J Neurosurg. 2003;98:1255–62.
51. Mikuni N, Okada T, Taki J, Matsumoto R, Nishida N, Enatsu R, et al. Fibers from the dorsal premotor cortex elicit motor-evoked potential in a cortical dysplasia. NeuroImage. 2007;34:12–8.
52. Kim CH, Chung CK, Lee SK, Lee YK, Chi JG. Parietal lobe epilepsy: surgical treatment and outcome. Stereotact Funct Neurosurg. 2004;82:175–85.
53. Sahjpaul RL. Awake craniotomy: controversies, indications and techniques in the surgical treatment of temporal lobe epilepsy. Can J Neurol Sci. 2000;27:S55–63.
54. Cohen-Gadol AA, Ozduman K, Bronen RA, Kim JH, Spencer DD. Long-term outcome after epilepsy surgery for focal cortical dysplasia. J Neurosurg. 2004;101:55–65.
55. Duffau H. Brain plasticity and tumors. Adv Tech Stand Neurosurg. 2008;3:3–33.
56. Duffau H. Lessons from brain mapping in surgery for low-grade glioma: insights into associations between tumour and brain plasticity. Lancet Neurol. 2005;4:476–86.
57. Duffau H. New concepts in surgery of WHO grade II gliomas: functional brain mapping, connectionism and plasticity – a review. J Neuro-Oncol. 2006;79:77–115.
58. Berger MS, Rostomily RC. Low grade gliomas: functional mapping resection strategies, extent of resection, and outcome. J Neuro Oncol. 1997;34:85–101.
59. Berger MS. Surgery of low-grade gliomas – technical aspects. Clin Neurosurg. 1997;44:161–80.
60. Ojemann JG, Miller JW, Silbergeld DL. Preserved function in brain invaded by tumor. Neurosurgery. 1996;39:253–8.
61. Ojemann JG, Ojemann GA, Lettich E. Cortical stimulation mapping of language cortex by using a verb generation task: effects of learning and comparison to mapping based on object naming. J Neurosurg. 2002;97:33–8.
62. Haglund MM, Berger MS, Shamseldin M, Lettich E, Ojemann GA. Cortical localization of temporal lobe language sites in patients with gliomas. Neurosurgery. 1994;34:567–76.
63. Duffau H, Lopes M, Arthuis F, Bitar A, Sichez JP, Van Effenterre R, et al. Contribution of intraoperative electrical stimulations in surgery of low grade gliomas: a comparative study between two series without (1985–96) and with (1996–2003) functional mapping in the same institution. J Neurol Neurosurg Psychiatry. 2005;76:845–51.
64. Pallud J, Mandonnet E, Duffau H, Kujas M, Guillevin R, Galanaud D, et al. Prognostic value of initial magnetic resonance imaging growth rates for World Health Organization grade II gliomas. Ann Neurol. 2006;60:380–3.
65. Desmurget M, Bonnetblanc F, Duffau H. Contrasting acute and slow-growing lesions: a new door to brain plasticity. Brain. 2007;130:898–914.
66. Duffau H, Taillandier L, Gatignol P, Capelle L. The insular lobe and brain plasticity: lessons from tumor surgery. Clin Neurol Neurosurg. 2006;108:543–8.
67. Burneo JG, Kuzniecky RI, Bebin M, Knowlton RC. Cortical reorganization in malformations of cortical development: a magnetoencephalographic study. Neurology. 2004;63:1818–24.
68. Coleshill SG, Binnie CD, Morris RG, et al. Material-specific recognition memory deficits elicited by unilateral hippocampal electrical stimulation. J Neurosci. 2004;24:1612–6.
69. Lacruz ME, Valentín A, Seoane JJ, Morris RG, Selway RP, Alarcón G. Single pulse electrical stimulation of the hippocampus is sufficient to impair human episodic memory. Neuroscience. 2010;170:623–32.
70. Tani N, Kishima H, Khoo HM, et al. Electrical stimulation of the parahippocampal gyrus for prediction of posthippocampectomy verbal memory decline. J Neurosurg. 2016;125:1053–60.
71. Kho KH, Rutten GJ, Leijten FS, van der Schaaf A, van Rijen PC, Ramsey NF. Working memory deficits after resection of the dorsolateral prefrontal cortex predicted by functional magnetic resonance imaging and electrocortical stimulation mapping. Case report. J Neurosurg. 2007;106:501–5.

72. Matsui Y, Maesawa S, Futamura M, Tobinaga M, Fujii M. Challenging for preservation of higher cognitive functions during awake surgery—a case demonstrating the association of attention in the dorsolateral prefrontal cortex in dominant hemisphere. Hr Brain Funct Res. 2015;35:1–8. (Japanese)
73. Duffau H, Capelle L, Sichez J, Faillot T, Abdennour L, Law Koune JD, et al. Intra-operative direct electrical stimulations of the central nervous system: the salpêtrière experience with 60 patients. Acta Neurochir. 1999;141:1157–67.
74. Duffau H. The reliability of asleep-awake-asleep protocol for intraoperative functional mapping and cognitive monitoring in glioma surgery. Acta Neurochir. 2013;155:1803–4.
75. Ghazanwy M, Chakrabarti R, Tewari A, Sinha A. Awake craniotomy: a qualitative review and future challenges. Saudi J Anaesth. 2014;8:529–39.
76. Stevanovic A, Rossaint R, Veldeman M, Bilotta F, Coburn M. Anaesthesia management for awake craniotomy: systematic review and meta-analysis. PLoS One. 2016;11:e0156448.
77. Andersen JH, Olsen KS. Anaesthesia for awake craniotomy is safe and well-tolerated. Dan Med Bull. 2010;57:A4194.
78. Chacko AG, Thomas SG, Babu KS, Daniel RT, Chacko G, Prabhu K, et al. Awake craniotomy and electrophysiological mapping for eloquent area tumours. Clin Neurol Neurosurg. 2013;115:329–34.
79. Gupta DK, Chandra PS, Ojha BK, Sharma BS, Mahapatra AK, Mehta VS, et al. Awake craniotomy versus surgery under general anesthesia for resection of intrinsic lesions of eloquent cortex – a prospective randomized study. Clin Neurol Neurosurg. 2007;109:335–43.
80. Hervey-Jumper SL, Li J, Lau D, Molinaro AM, Perry DW, Meng L, et al. Awake craniotomy to maximize glioma resection: methods and technical nuances over a 27-year period. J Neurosurg. 2015;123:325–39.
81. Shinoura N, Midorikawa A, Yamada R, Hana T, Saito A, Hiromitsu K, et al. Awake craniotomy for brain lesions within and near the primary motor area: a retrospective analysis of factors associated with worsened paresis in 102 consecutive patients. Surg Neurol Int. 2013;4:149.
82. Nossek E, Matot I, Shahar T, Barzilai O, Rapoport Y, Gonen T, et al. Intraoperative seizures during awake craniotomy: incidence and consequences: analysis of 477 patients. Neurosurgery. 2013;73:135–40.
83. Li T, Bai H, Wang G, Wang W, Lin J, Gao H, et al. Glioma localization and excision using direct electrical stimulation for language mapping during awake surgery. Exp Ther Med. 2015;9:1962–6.
84. Souter MJ, Rozet I, Ojemann JG, Souter KJ, Holmes MD, Lee L, et al. Dexmedetomidine sedation during awake craniotomy for seizure resection: effects on electrocorticography. J Neurosurg Anesthesiol. 2007;19:38–44.
85. Mahmoud M, Sadhasivam S, Salisbury S, Nick TG, Schnell B, Sestokas AK, et al. Susceptibility of transcranial electric motor-evoked potentials to varying targeted blood levels of dexmedetomidine during spine surgery. Anesthesiology. 2010;112:1364–73.
86. Pillai S, Hoehn K, Brouillette G. Posterior reversible encephalopathy syndrome as a result of withdrawal from prolonged dexmedetomidine. J Pediatr Intensive Care. 2015;4:162–5.
87. McNicholas E, Bilotta F, Titi L, Chandler J, Rosa G, Koht A, et al. Transient facial nerve palsy after auriculotemporal nerve block in awake craniotomy patients. A A Case Rep. 2014;2:40–3.
88. Osborn I, Sebeo J. "Scalp block" during craniotomy: a classic technique revisited. J Neurosurg Anesthesiol. 2010;22:187–94.
89. Guilfoyle MR, Helmy A, Duane D, Hutchinson PJ. Regional scalp block for postcraniotomy analgesia: a systematic review and meta-analysis. Anesth Analg. 2013;116:1093–102.
90. Sidhu A, Murgahayah T, Narayanan V, Chandran H, Waran V. Electroacupuncture-assisted craniotomy on an awake patient. J Acupunct Meridian Stud. 2017;10:45–8.
91. Krsek P, Maton B, Jayakar P, et al. Incomplete resection of focal cortical dysplasia is the main predictor of poor postsurgical outcome. Neurology. 2009;72:217–23.
92. Chang EF, Wang DD, Barkovich AJ, et al. Predictors of seizure freedom after surgery for malformations of cortical development. Ann Neurol. 2011;70:151–62.
93. Fernández IS, Loddenkemper T. Electrocorticography for seizure foci mapping in epilepsy surgery. J Clin Neurophysiol. 2013;30:554–70.
94. Wyllie E, Lüders H, Morris HH, et al. Clinical outcome after complete or partial cortical resection for intractable epilepsy. Neurology. 1987;37:1634–41.
95. Asano E, Juhász C, Shah A, Sood S, Chugani HT. Role of subdural electrocorticography in prediction of long-term seizure outcome in epilepsy surgery. Brain. 2009;132:1038–47.
96. Benifla M, Otsubo H, Ochi A, et al. Temporal lobe surgery for intractable epilepsy in children: an analysis of outcomes in 126 children. Neurosurgery. 2006;59:1203–13; discussion 1213–4.
97. McKhann GM, Schoenfeld-McNeill J, Born DE, Haglund MM, Ojemann GA. Intraoperative hippocampal electrocorticography to predict the extent of hippocampal resection in temporal lobe epilepsy surgery. J Neurosurg. 2000;93:44–52.
98. Hosain S, Burton L, Fraser R, Labar D. Focal suppression-burst on electrocorticography after temporal lobectomy. Neurology. 1995;45:2276–8.
99. Schwartz TH, Bazil CW, Forgione M, Bruce JN, Goodman RR. Do reactive post-resection "injury" spikes exist? Epilepsia. 2000;41:1463–8.
100. Rasmussen T. Characteristics of a pure culture of frontal lobe epilepsy. Epilepsia. 1983;24:482–93.
101. Jacobs J, LeVan P, Chander R, Hall J, Dubeau F, Gotman J. Interictal high-frequency oscillations

(80-500 Hz) are an indicator of seizure onset areas independent of spikes in the human epileptic brain. Epilepsia. 2008;49:1893–907.
102. Wu JY, Sankar R, Lerner JT, Matsumoto JH, Vinters HV, Mathern GW. Removing interictal fast ripples on electrocorticography linked with seizure freedom in children. Neurology. 2010;75:1686–94.
103. Urrestarazu E, Chander R, Dubeau F, Gotman J. Interictal high-frequency oscillations (100-500 Hz) in the intracerebral EEG of epileptic patients. Brain. 2007;130:2354–66.
104. Andrade-Valença L, Mari F, Jacobs J, et al. Interictal high frequency oscillations (HFOs) in patients with focal epilepsy and normal MRI. Clin Neurophysiol. 2012;123:100–5.
105. Asano E, Benedek K, Shah A, et al. Is intraoperative electrocorticography reliable in children with intractable neocortical epilepsy? Epilepsia. 2004;45:1091–9.
106. Morsy AA, Ismail AM, Nasr YM, Waly SH, Abdelhameed EA. Predictors of stimulation-induced seizures during perirolandic glioma resection using intraoperative mapping techniques. Surg Neurol Int. 2021;12:117.
107. Nossek E, Matot I, Shahar T, Barzilai O, Rapoport Y, Gonen T, Sela G, Grossman R, Korn A, Hayat D, Ram Z. Intraoperative seizures during awake craniotomy: incidence and consequences - analysis of 477 patients. Neurosurgery. 2013;73:135. https://doi.org/10.1227/01.neu.0000429847.91707.97.
108. Chakraborty A, McEvoy AW. Presurgical functional mapping with functional MRI. Curr Opin Neurol. 2008;21(4):446–51.
109. Rolinski R, Austermuehle A, Wiggs E, Agrawal S, Leigh N, Gaillard W. Functional MRI and direct cortical stimulation: prediction of postoperative language decline. Epilepsia. 2019;60:560–70.
110. Gil Robles S, Gelisse P, Vergani F, Moritz-Gasser S, Rigau V, Coubes P, et al. Discrepancies between preoperative stereoencephalography language stimulation mapping and intraoperative awake mapping during resection of focal cortical dysplasia in eloquent areas. Stereotact Funct Neurosurg. 2008;86(6):382–90.
111. Vincent M, Rossel O, Duffau H, et al. A measure of cortico-cortical potentials evoked by 10 Hz direct electrical stimulation of the brain and by means of a differential recording mode of electrocorticographic signals. Conf Proc IEEE Eng Med Biol Soc. 2016;2016:4543–6.

Patient Selection for Awake Craniotomy <Patient Selection, Awake Craniotomy>

Mehmet Erdal Coşkun and Fatih Yakar

1 Introduction

The first awake craniotomy (AC) applications were found in archaeological excavations in Peru. The successful healing rate was 55% of trephinations in 214 skulls. Coca leaves were used as a local anesthetic before the general anesthesia (GA) era. The first recorded case of AC was the epilepsy surgery performed by Sir Victor Horsley in 1886 [1]. He resected an epileptogenic lesion from a 22-year-old man. Wilder Penfield popularized the procedure in the first half of the twentieth century [2]. Compared with GA, AC has the following advantages after tumor resection: improved outcome; greater extent of tumor resection; fewer late neurological deficits, and shorter hospital stay [3–5].

The main indication for AC has been in patients with tumors adjacent to eloquent (i.e., motor, sensory, language, or cognitive functions) brain areas [6]. Moreover, AC has been adopted as a standard approach in some centers to reduce the risk of additional morbidity caused by GA and intubation in patients with low Karnofksy performance status (KPS) scores [7, 8].

Improvements in anesthetic care have contributed significantly to the development of AC [5]. There are two variants of AC: the asleep-awake-asleep procedure, in which the patient is awake during cortical mapping and tumor resection; and the monitored anesthesia care procedure, in which the patient is awake during the entire operation [9].

Although the success of AC mainly depends on the correct patient selection, there are no standardized criteria in the literature. The Japan Awake Surgery Conference (established in 2002) prepared a guideline for AC in 2012 [8] and it is the only guideline in the current literature. This guideline consists of three main headings: surgical maneuvers, anesthetic management, and language assessment. In each sub-heading, a recommendation was given first and then referenced articles were added and discussed. This attempt to standardize the AC procedure has not yet gained international acceptance. In this chapter, we determined the patient and lesion-related factors that should be evaluated in the preoperative period and have suggested what could contribute to appropriate patient selection for AC.

2 Patient-Related Factors

Although the essential requirement for AC is the patient's volunteerism [10], factors such as mental status, seizure history, antiepileptic drug (AED) use, pregnancy, age weight, and preoperative neurological function will be evaluated in this section. To reduce anxiety, the patient can be

M. E. Coşkun (✉) · F. Yakar
Department of Neurosurgery, Pamukkale University School of Medicine, Denizli, Turkey
e-mail: e.coskun@iku.edu.tr

A. Pour-Rashidi, J. Aarabi (eds.), *The Principles of Successful Awake Craniotomy*,
https://doi.org/10.1007/978-981-99-2985-6_4

taken to the operating room the day before surgery. The location of the surgical and anesthesia team during the operation should also be explained. The position during the operation can be demonstrated to the patient and practiced encouraging patient compliance. Unlike in sleep surgeries, during awake surgeries, patients may have to tolerate some discomfort related to body positions and pain caused by head immobilization, incisions, airway protection, and nausea [11].

The procedure should be explained to the patient with videos before the surgery. Details are articulated concerning which stage the pain may occur and what is expected from the patient during that process. Situations requiring GA are explained to the patient and informed consent should be signed. Overall, patient rejection is probably the only nonsurgical contraindication for AC.

2.1 Mental/Neurologic Status and Post-traumatic Stress Disorder (PTSD)

The success of AC depends on the patient's mental state and cooperation. For this procedure, the patient's mental health [12–14] and cognition performance [14] must be assessed sufficiently. The psychological evaluation is assessed with Mini Mental State Scale [14]. The cognitive level is assessed with Addenbrooke's Cognitive Examination (ACE III) the day before surgery. With ACE III, five domains are evaluated out of 100 points: attention/ orientation (18 points); memory (26 points); word fluency (14 points); language (26 points); and visuospatial functions (16 points). The sensitivity and specificity cutoff values for mild cognitive impairment in ACE III are 88 and 82, respectively [15].

Some authors consider anxiety disorders an obstacle to AC [16, 17]. The Anxiety Scale of the Dutch version of the Hospital Anxiety and Depression Scale is a test with seven questions and a maximum score of 21 used to measure the preoperative anxiety level [18]. The expressions to be scored on this scale are as follows: "I feel tense" or "wound up"; "I get a sort of frightened feeling as if something awful is about to happen"; "worrying thoughts go through my mind"; "I can sit at ease and feel relaxed"; "I get a sort of frightened feeling like 'butterflies' in the stomach"; " I feel restless as I have to be on the move and I get sudden feelings of panic." Each statement is scored between 0 and 3 points. Above 7 points are the most optimal sensitivity and specificity as a case finder for anxiety disorders [19].

In the presence of a multidisciplinary approach, rigorous preoperative evaluation, patient education, and a controlled intraoperative environment, PTSD was not considered an exclusion criterion [20, 21].

Patients with severe aphasia have been excluded from many studies [13]. If the patient has already developed moderate or severe symptoms, mapping and monitoring will be difficult. Patients with impairment in understanding, reading, repetition, and object naming are not suitable candidates for AC. Patients who cannot speak fluently but whose understanding and naming are not impaired are suitable for AC [22].

The recommendation of the Japan Awake Surgery Conference guideline [8] suggests that patient participation is essential in AC along with the surgical team so that everyone understands the meaning of aggressive tumor resection and possible complications. The surgical team should be aware of whether or not the patient can tolerate AC.

2.2 Seizure and Antiepileptic Drug Use History

It can be said that seizure occurrence at onset and intractable epilepsy do not increase the risk of intraoperative seizures (IOS) [23]. In contrast, some studies have found a correlation between preoperative seizures and IOS [5, 24, 25]. Multiple AEDs used for the preexistence of intractable epilepsy were found not to affect IOS [5, 24, 26]. The effects of prophylactic AED use on seizure-free patients remain controversial. A recent multicenter study [25] found no impact of prophylactic AED on IOS.

The anterior areas (frontal, supplementary motor area, and premotor cortex) are associated with a higher risk for IOS [24, 27]. The intrinsic epileptogenicity is usually higher for World Health Organization (WHO) grade II gliomas [28].

The recommendation of the Japan Awake Surgery Conference guideline [8] states that patients who are scheduled for AC, if there is enough time, antiepileptic treatment should be started to reach adequate blood levels. Phenytoin can be administered and the target level to be reached the day before surgery is 20 mg/dl. Phenytoin is recommended because there are both oral and intravenous forms of this drug. In addition, it takes 4–5 days to reach a sufficient level in the blood and concentration is easy to control. Especially in lesions close to the motor cortex, after reaching the appropriate drug concentration in the blood, the drug level should be checked every 2 h in surgery. During surgery, if the concentration is low, 250 mg of phenytoin is given intravenously (which increases drug concentration to 6 mg/dl in a 60 kg patient) or 100–200 mg of phenytoin every 4 h (which increases drug concentration to 2.4–4.7 mg/dl in a 60 kg patient).

2.3 Pregnancy

Tumor occurrence in pregnancy is extremely rare and treatment planning becomes difficult in these cases. While the neurosurgical approach is typically delayed after fetal delivery in neurologically stable patients, urgent tumor resection is required in neurologically unstable patients [29]. If fetal distress develops during AC, emergency cesarean section is performed with epidural anesthesia or GA. It may also be a good option to initiate the case with an epidural catheter [30].

AC procedure was reported to have been successfully performed in some eloquent area lesions during pregnancy [30–32]; however, since there are no large case series on this subject, it is not possible to make a clear assessment.

2.4 Age

Pediatric populations present special challenges, such as difficulties with cooperation, understanding, and managing co-occurring anxiety [33]. Although AC has well-documented benefits, it was stated in a recent review that AC remains mainly limited to adults since there is no guideline for standardization in the pediatric age group; however, AC was reported to be safe in selected patient groups [34]. In the pediatric population, a psychological/neuropsychological assessment and preparation for a preoperative eligibility assessment and a final eligibility decision are obligatory. During the surgical procedure, psychological/neuropsychological support should be offered by a familiar professional who provides the initial assessment and preparation. Finally, psychological/neuropsychological follow-up is recommended at ages 3, 6, and 12 months postoperatively [34].

In many studies, the age criteria for inclusion is over 18 years [13] but some AC series include patients in the pediatric age group [7, 35–38]. Pasquet [39] stated that uncooperative adults and children under 10 years will not tolerate local anesthesia, scalp incision, and craniotomy and defined the age limit as ten. The youngest patient who underwent AC in the literature is 8 years old [40]. It is difficult to stimulate the cortex with electrical stimulation in the patient group aged 7 years and younger. Moreover, this age group does not meet the criteria for cortical electrical stimulation [22]. In a study involving patients over 18 years of age, it was found that the level of psychological trauma and PTSD was not clinically apparent [13]. In contrast, Klimek et al. [37] stated that it seemed unacceptable to set an age restriction and suitability for surgery should be determined by the individual developmental level of the child.

The recommendation of the Japan Awake Surgery Conference guideline [8] stated that each patient should be carefully evaluated by the anesthesiologist, surgeon, and language therapist, and there is no specific upper age limit. Surgeons with limited AC experience should try this surgery on patients aged 15–65 years.

2.5 Weight

Morbidly obese patients are not ideal candidates for AC. Airway obstruction, collapse, obstructive sleep apnea, sensitivity to anesthetics, and sedations were reported more frequently in this patient group. Since airway management is more difficult in these patients during possible surgical complications (e.g., seizure, stroke), the rate of conversion to GA and the rate of patients not benefiting from AC is higher. Airway collapse could be prevented with the help of heated humidified high-flow nasal cannula oxygen therapy [41, 42]. There is no consensus on obesity as some publications reflect that obesity is contraindicated for AC [10], while other researchers differ in opinion concerning AC [43].

2.6 Preoperative KPS Score

The neurological function evaluation is conducted by using the KPS score. We preferred AC particularly in our series [7] in patients with a preoperative KPS score of less than 100. The main purpose for choosing AC in patients with low KPS scores was to avoid additional morbidities that may be caused by GA. However, there is no clear information in the literature between KPS score and AC indication. Furthermore, patients with severely compromised heart, lung, liver, and kidney function were excluded from most studies [14].

2.7 Other Unspecified Conditions

Movement disorders, inability to lie flat/still for a prolonged period, severe gastric reflux [10], claustrophobia, mood instability, apparent dysphagia, alcohol, or drug dependence, chronic pain disorders, restless leg syndrome, low pain tolerance, obstructive sleep apnea, and uncontrolled cough are reported relative contraindications for AC [44]. The awake (or with minimal sedation) deep brain stimulation was historically approved for Parkinson's disease, essential tremor, and dystonia. Therefore, movement disorders are considered a relative contraindication.

3 Lesion-Related Factors

The location, size, number, and pathology of the lesion in the intracranial space can be evaluated as lesion-related factors. These factors may cause seizures and increased intracranial pressure (ICP). Compared to patient-related factors, lesion-related factors are less effective in patient selection for AC.

3.1 Location

Although Berger [36], reported that AC in the occipital lobe was contraindicated in the previous decades, AC can be safely applied in all supratentorial areas today [6]. In addition, deeply located lesions such as the insula, corpus callosum, and thalamus in the supratentorial area are not contraindicated to AC [6]. There are also studies on the application of AC in the infratentorial area [45, 46].

In our experience [7] in ventricular surgery. nausea and vomiting may occur when the surgeon enters the ventricles. The necessity of antiemetic therapy should be considered before entering the ventricle. Skull-base and falx dura are sensitive to pain (in the sensory territories of the V1 and V3 divisions of the trigeminal nerve) [47]. Therefore, pain control should be provided at an optimum level during dura opening.

There is a risk of air embolism in tumors of the motor cortex since the surgical field will be at its highest point. In this patient group, we need to bend the head toward the ground in the sagittal plane first along with elevating the lower extremity that increases jugular venous pressure. After opening the skull, the skull should be covered with fibrin, thrombin, and calciol. The head should be kept down until the dura is opened, and then the head should be raised gradually, following SaO_2. If there are symptoms such as cough and a decrease in SaO_2 and cough, the head should be put down and the neck should be supported [48].

The recommendation of the Japan Awake Surgery Conference guideline [8] for tumor sites states that the lateral parietal lobe of the dominant hemisphere (mainly including the angular gyrus), lesions adjacent to arcuate fibers (superior longitudinal fasciculus), motor cortex, the triangular and opercular regions of the posterior part of the inferior frontal gyrus (Brodmann's areas 44 and 45), inferior part of the precentral gyrus with respect to the language motor center, in the posterior half of the superior, middle and inferior temporal gyri of the temporal lobe (areas 41, 42, 22, and 37), and supramarginal gyrus (area 40) with respect to sensory language center and hippocampus can be considered for awake surgery.

3.2 Size and Multiplicity of the Lesion

Although Dziedzic and Bernstein [49] stated that GA would be more accurate in large tumors, they did not specify a precise size. We did not consider tumor size a contraindication in our clinical series [7] and did not find any contraindication related to tumor size in other recent studies. Multiplicity was not considered a contraindication in the literature [6].

3.3 Pathology

Brain tumor removal, epilepsy surgery, deep brain stimulation, and endarterectomy are the main procedures for AC [50, 51]. Patients with low-grade gliomas, high-grade gliomas, metastasis, cavernomas, intra-axial epidermoid cysts, meningiomas, abscess, radiation necrosis, and lymphoma underwent AC in the literature review [6, 52]. AC is also applied in vestibular schwannomas [53], microvascular decompression for trigeminal neuralgia [54], aneurysms [55], bypass surgery [56], and arteriovenous malformations (AVM) [57, 58]. From a neurosurgical perspective, the use of GA is preferred in highly vascular tumors as well as in cases where blood loss will be high since patient cooperation may be impaired [49].

The recommendation of the Japan Awake Surgery Conference guideline [8] for ICP is Arterial carbon dioxide tension ($PaCO_2$) tends to be higher in AC than in GA and may increase ICP. GA should be preferred if there are signs of increased ICP in preoperative imaging. However, if AC is absolutely necessary, the decision can be made after standard intubation followed by a dural incision. If there is swelling in the brain, continue with GA, but if there is no swelling, it can be switched to AC after extubation.

4 Conclusion

There is little consensus on indications and contraindications for AC. There are dozens of patients or lesion-related factors, where one surgeon may suggest AC while another may state that it is contraindicated. During the preoperative period, the patient should have a full understanding of what is expected during surgery; and the operating process is explained to the patient in the operating room with or without video presentation, to reduce the level of patient anxiety. The patient's compliance, volunteerism, and multidisciplinary approach are the keys to success in the AC procedure.

References

1. Horsley V. Remarks on ten consecutive cases of operations upon the brain and cranial cavity to illustrate the details and safety of the method employed. Br Med J. 1887;1:863–5.
2. Penfield W, Boldrey E. Somatic motor and sensory representation in the cerebral cortex of man as studied by electrical stimulation. Brain. 1937;60:3890443.
3. De Witt Hamer PC, Robles SG, Zwinderman AH, et al. Impact of intraoperative stimulation brain mapping on glioma surgery outcome: a meta-analysis. J Clin Oncol. 2012;30:2559–65.
4. Sacko O, Lauwers-Cances V, Brauge D, et al. Awake craniotomy vs surgery under general anesthesia for resection of supratentorial lesions. Neurosurgery. 2011;68:1192–8.
5. Hervey-Jumper SL, Li J, Lau D, et al. Awake craniotomy to maximize glioma resection: methods and technical nuances over a 27-year period. J Neurosurg. 2015;123(2):325–39.

6. Takami H, Khoshnood N, Bernstein M. Preoperative factors associated with adverse events during awake craniotomy: analysis of 609 consecutive cases. J Neurosurg. 2020;134(5):1631–9.
7. Coskun E, Yakar F, Civlan S, et al. Experience of fully awake craniotomy for supratentorial lesions: a single institution study. Turk Neurosurg. 2020;30(6):907–13.
8. Kayama T. Guidelines committee of the Japan awake surgery conference. The guidelines for awake craniotomy guidelines committee of the Japan awake surgery conference. Neurol Med Chir (Tokyo). 2012;52(3):119–41.
9. Duffau H. Jazz improvisation, creativity, and brain plasticity. World Neurosurgery. 2014;81(3–4):508–10.
10. Hill CS, Severgnini F, McKintosh E. How I do it: awake craniotomy. Acta Neurochir (Wien). 2017;159(1):173–6.
11. Conte V, Baratta P, Tomaselli P, et al. Awake neurosurgery: an update. Minerva Anestesiol. 2008;74(6):289–92.
12. Chouhan RS, Khandelwal A, Biswas K, et al. Awake craniotomy during menstruation: is it advisable? Neurol India. 2020;68(2):493–4.
13. Starowicz-Filip A, Prochwicz K, Myszka A, et al. Subjective experience, cognitive functioning and trauma level of patients undergoing awake craniotomy due to brain tumor - preliminary study. Appl Neuropsychol Adult. 2022;29:983. https://doi.org/10.1080/23279095.2020.1831500.
14. Chen X, Sun J, Jiang W, et al. Awake craniotomy for removal of gliomas in eloquent areas: an analysis of 21 cases. Brain Res Bull. 2022;181:30–5.
15. Velayudhan L, Seung-Ho R, Raczek M, et al. Review of brief cognitive tests for patients with suspected dementia. Int Psychogeriatr. 2014;26(8):1247–62.
16. Ruis C, Wajer IH, Robe P, et al. Anxiety in the preoperative phase of awake brain tumor surgery. Clin Neurol Neurosurg. 2017;157:7–10.
17. Santini B, Talacchi A, Casagrande F, et al. Eligibility criteria and psychological profiles in patient candidates for awake craniotomy: a pilot study. J Neurosurg Anesthesiol. 2012;24(3):209–16.
18. Zigmond AS, Snaith RP. The hospital anxiety and depression scale. Acta Psychiatr Scand. 1983;67(6):361–70.
19. Bjelland I, Dahl AA, Haug TT, et al. The validity of the Hospital Anxiety and Depression Scale. An updated literature review. J Psychosom Res. 2002;52(2):69–77.
20. Ma K, Uejima JL. Awake craniotomy in a patient with history of post-traumatic stress disorder-a clinical dilemma: a case report. A A Pract. 2020;14(5):140–3.
21. Marenco-Hillembrand L, Suarez-Meade P, Sabsevitz DS, et al. Awake craniotomy in a patient with previously diagnosed post-traumatic stress disorder. World Neurosurg. 2020;139:7–11.
22. Berger MS, Ojemann GA, Lettich E. Neurophysiological monitoring during astrocytoma surgery. Neurosurg Clin N Am. 1990;1(1):65–80.
23. Yuan Y, Peizhi Z, Xiang W, et al. Intraoperative seizures and seizures outcome in patients undergoing awake craniotomy. J Neurosurg Sci. 2019;63(3):301–7.
24. Nossek E, Matot I, Shahar T, et al. Intraoperative seizures during awake craniotomy: incidence and consequences: analysis of 477 patients. Neurosurgery. 2013;73(01):135–40; discussion 140.
25. Spena G, Schucht P, Seidel K, et al. Brain tumors in eloquent areas: a European multicenter survey of intraoperative mapping techniques, intraoperative seizures occurrence, and antiepileptic drug prophylaxis. Neurosurg Rev. 2017;40(2):287–98.
26. Boetto J, Bertram L, Moulinié G, et al. Low rate of intraoperative seizures during awake craniotomy in a prospective cohort with 374 supratentorial brain lesions: electrocorticography is not mandatory. World Neurosurg. 2015;84(06):1838–44.
27. Gonen T, Grossman R, Sitt R, et al. Tumor location and IDH1 mutation may predict intraoperative seizures during awake craniotomy. J Neurosurg. 2014;121(05):1133–8.
28. Pallud J, Le Van QM, Bielle F, et al. Cortical GABAergic excitation contributes to epileptic activities around human glioma. Sci Transl Med. 2014;6(244):244ra89.
29. Tewari KS, Cappuccini F, Asrat T, et al. Obstetric emergencies precipitated by malignant brain tumors. Am J Obstet Gynecol. 2000;182:1215–21.
30. Meng L, Han SJ, Rollins MD, et al. Awake brain tumor resection during pregnancy: decision making and technical nuances. J Clin Neurosci. 2016;24:160–2.
31. Handlogten KS, Sharpe EE, Brost BC, et al. Dexmedetomidine and mannitol for awake craniotomy in a pregnant patient. Anesth Analg. 2015;120(5):1099–103.
32. Al Mashani AM, Ali A, Chatterjee N, et al. Awake craniotomy during pregnancy. J Neurosurg Anesthesiol. 2018;30(4):372–3.
33. Everett LL, van Rooyen IF, Warner MH, et al. Use of dexmedetomidine in awake craniotomy in adolescents: report of two cases. Paediatr Anaesth. 2006;16:338–42.
34. Lohkamp LN, Mottolese C, Szathmari A, et al. Awake brain surgery in children-review of the literature and state-of-the-art. Childs Nerv Syst. 2019;35(11):2071–7.
35. Alcaraz García-Tejedor G, Echániz G, Strantzas S, et al. Feasibility of awake craniotomy in the pediatric population. Paediatr Anaesth. 2020;30(4):480–9.
36. Berger MS. The impact of technical adjuncts in the surgical management of cerebral hemispheric low-grade gliomas of childhood. J Neurooncol. 1996;28:129–55.
37. Klimek M, Verbrugge SJC, Roubos S, et al. Awake craniotomy for glioblastoma in a 9-year-old child. Anaesthesia. 2004;59(6):607–9.
38. Prabhakar H, Mahajan C, Kapoor I. Awake craniotomy in pediatric population is possible! Paediatr Anaesth. 2020;30(6):722.

39. Pasquet A. Combine regional and general anesthesia for craniotomy and cortical exploration. Part II. Anesthetic considerations. Anesth Analg. 1954;33:156–7.
40. Riquin E, Dinomais M, Malka J, et al. Psychiatric and psychological impact of surgery while awake in children for resection of brain tumors. World Neurosurg. 2017;102:400–5.
41. Mahajan C, Rath GP, Singh GP, et al. Efficacy and safety of dexmedetomidine infusion for patients undergoing awake craniotomy: an observational study. Saudi J Anaesth. 2018;12:235–9.
42. Smith SC, Burbridge M, Jaffe R. High flow nasal cannula, a novel approach to airway management in awake craniotomies. J Neurosurg Anesthesiol. 2018;30:382.
43. Banik S, Parrent AG, Noppens RR. Awake craniotomy in a super obese patient using high flow nasal cannula oxygen therapy (HFNC). Anaesthesist. 2019;68(11):780–3.
44. Venkatraghavan L, Pasternak JJ, Crowley M. Anesthesia for awake craniotomy [UpToDate web site]. https://www.uptodate.com/contents/anesthesia-for-awakecraniotomy/print Accessed 20 Nov 2017.
45. Deipolyi AR, Han SJ, Sughrue ME, et al. Awake far lateral craniotomy for resection of foramen magnum meningioma in a patient with tenuous motor and somatosensory evoked potentials. J Clin Neurosci. 2011;18(9):1254–6.
46. Pereira EA, Jegan T, Green AL. Awake stereotactic brainstem biopsy via a contralateral, transfrontal, transventricular approach. Br J Neurosurg. 2008;22(4):599–601.
47. Fontaine D, Almairac F, Santucci S, et al. Dural and pial pain-sensitive structures in humans: new inputs from awake craniotomies. Brain. 2018;141(4):1040–8.
48. Scuplak SM, Smith M, Harkness WF. Air embolism during awake craniotomy. Anaesthesia. 1995;50(4):338–40.
49. Dziedzic T, Bernstein M. Awake craniotomy for brain tumor: indications, technique and benefits. Expert Rev Neurother. 2014;14:1405–15.
50. Dreier JD, Williams B, Mangar D, et al. Patients selection for awake neurosurgery. HSR Proc Intensive Care Cardiovasc Anesth. 2009;1(4):19–27.
51. Serletis D, Bernstein M. Prospective study of awake craniotomy used routinely and nonselectively for supratentorial tumors. J Neurosurg. 2007;107(1):1–6.
52. Albuquerque LAF, Diógenes GS, Pessoa FC. Challenges in starting an awake craniotomy project in a low-resource public health system. World Neurosurg. 2021;146:277–9.
53. Shinoura N, Midorikawa A, Hiromitsu K, et al. Preservation of hearing following awake surgery via the retrosigmoid approach for vestibular schwannomas in eight consecutive patients. Acta Neurochir (Wien). 2017;159(9):1579–85.
54. Abdulrauf SI, Urquiaga JF, Patel R, et al. Awake microvascular decompression for trigeminal neuralgia: concept and initial results. World Neurosurg. 2018;113:e309–13.
55. Cannizzaro D, Peschillo S, Mancarella C, et al. Clipping in awake surgery as end-stage in a complex internal carotid artery aneurysm after failure of multimodal endovascular and extracranial-intracranial bypass treatment. J Stroke Cerebrovasc Dis. 2017;26(6):e114–8.
56. Abdulrauf SI, Urquiaga JF, Patel R, et al. Awake high-flow extracranial to intracranial bypass for complex cerebral aneurysms: institutional clinical trial results. World Neurosurg. 2017;105:557–67.
57. Ménissier A, Petit A, Bougaci N, et al. Interest of awake surgery for ruptured cerebral arteriovenous malformations close to speech areas - surgical note. Neurochirurgie. 2022;68:320. https://doi.org/10.1016/j.neuchi.2021.06.005.
58. Richter KR, Turcotte EL, Hess RA, et al. Awake resection of an arteriovenous malformation. World Neurosurg. 2021;162:17. https://doi.org/10.1016/j.wneu.2021.06.146.

Preoperative Conventional and Advanced Neuroimaging for Awake Craniotomy <Conventional Neuroimaging, Advanced Neuroimaging, Preoperative Neuroimaging>

Samira Raminfard and Mohsen Izanlou

1 Introduction

Neuroimaging noninvasively provides valuable information about brain structure, physiology, and function. Since the discovery of magnetic resonance imaging (MRI), it has played an efficient role in the diagnosis, treatment planning, and follow-up assessment of brain lesions. Conventional neuroimaging is used to evaluate the lesion location, extension to periphery, size, and effect upon the ventricular and vascular system. Advanced neuroimaging such as functional MRI (fMRI), diffusion tensor imaging (DTI), perfusion-weighted imaging (PWI), and magnetic resonance spectroscopy (MRS) has a more effective role to assess brain function, metabolism, and biochemical changes. In this chapter, we provide an overview of the current state of conventional and advanced neuroimaging protocols as it relates to presurgical planning for awake craniotomy.

S. Raminfard (✉)
Advanced Diagnostic and Interventional Radiology Research Center (ADIR), Tehran University of Medical Sciences, Tehran, Iran

Neuroimaging and Analysis Group (NIAG), Research Center for Molecular and Cellular Imaging, Advanced Medical Technologies and Equipment Institute, Tehran University of Medical Sciences, Tehran, Iran

M. Izanlou
Department of Radiology, Razi Hospital, Guilan University of Medical Sciences, Rasht, Iran

2 Conventional Brain Tumor Imaging

Current standard MRI protocol for brain lesions includes the following: T1-weighted image; fluid attenuation inversion recovery (FLAIR); T2-weighted image; diffusion-weighted imaging (DWI), and post-contrast T1. The primary role of conventional imaging is the evaluation of tumor location, tissue texture, size of tumor, and peripheral edema. Pre-contrast T1 images as an anatomical image are used for distinguishing suspicious bleeding as well as blood products, calcification, and fat [1]. Post-contrast imaging allows for appraisement of tumor vascularity and probability of blood–brain barrier (BBB) disruption. Enhancing lesions in glioma cases are positively correlated to malignancy of the tumor, although non-enhancing high-grade glioma has been reported [2]. The hyper-signal area in T2/FLAIR images refers to the mixture of edema and tumor core in non-enhancing lesions, so the tumor border is indistinguishable in such cases. In enhancing tumors, the T2/FLAIR hyperintense regions are known as vasogenic edema.

A. Pour-Rashidi, J. Aarabi (eds.), *The Principles of Successful Awake Craniotomy*,
https://doi.org/10.1007/978-981-99-2985-6_5

posterior frontal lobe (middle frontal gyrus and IFG), posterior two-thirds of temporal lobe (superior and middle temporal gyrus) [21]
- Meaning of words and sentences, semantic processing, distributed to multiple locations including the posterior and middle third of the superior and middle temporal gyrus, dorsolateral prefrontal cortex (DLPFC), and IFG [22]
- Rules for combination of words (syntax)

fMRI could inform us about the region of brain that corresponds to these modules [23]. Indeed, specific tasks should be applied during imaging to achieve the best result.

6 Language Paradigms

In a fMRI study, both visual and auditory cues were presented in the language tasks [24]. It has been reported that these two types of cues produced similar brain activation patterns [25]. To establish an effective protocol for language mapping, studies designed to determine which paradigm or combination of them provide adequate and valid localization in receptive and expressive language networks. In 2016, the American Society of Functional Neuroradiology (ASFN) reviewed different institute results for clinical fMRI and recommended fMRI paradigm for clinical language assessments. Based on their review, the default language algorithm is sentence completion, silent word generation, and rhyming. Below are some examples of frequently used tasks for clinical language fMRI.

6.1 Sentence Completion

During the active block of this task, sentences with the last word missing were presented and the patients were instructed to complete each sentence with a correct word. This verbal comprehension task is an effective evaluation task for activation in the superior temporal gyrus, and less robustly, can also activate expressive language area in dominant IFG [26] and the visual word form area via activation of the ventral language stream [27]. El Salek and collogues (2017), showed that "the silent sentence completion is a robust paradigm for localizing Wernicke's area" (Fig. 1) [28].

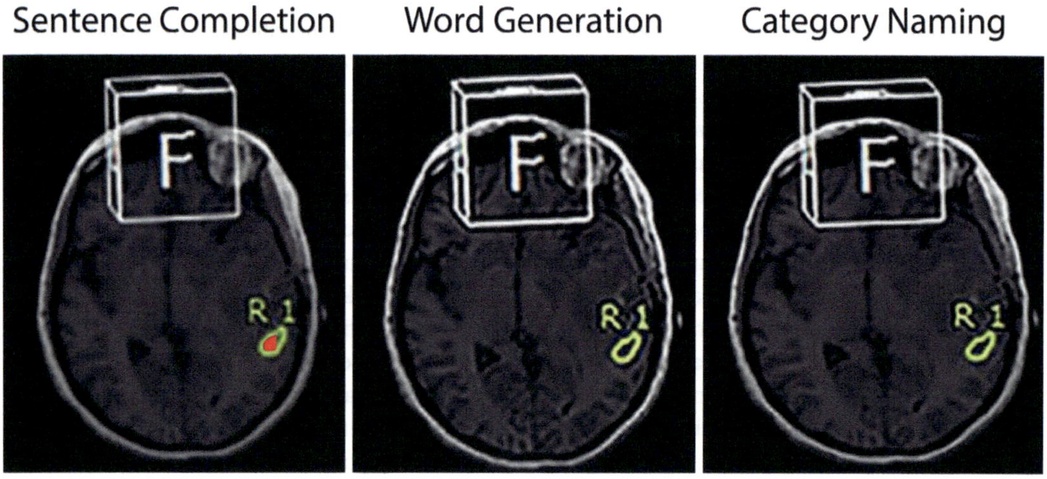

Fig. 1 ROI (yellow outline) at the location of Wernicke's area showing activity on Silent Sentence Completion, Verbal fluency (FAS), and Category Naming (CAT), from left to right, respectively in a patient with left temporal glioblastoma. SSC showed eight active voxels (red); no active voxels detected on FAS and CAT (No need to get permission) [28]

6.2 Silent Word Generation

In this task, patients were to generate as many words as possible from a given letter (e.g., book, bus, butter for b) or lexical category (e.g., animals, tools) [29–31]. In contrast to sentence completion task, silent word generation yielded reliable activation in IFG, DLPFC, superior frontal, and supplementary motor area (SMA) (Fig. 2) and less robust activation in the temporal cortex [32]. Zaca et al. (2013) revealed that the word generation was the best paradigm for localization of expressive area in frontal lobe. The combination of this verbal fluency practice with other semantic paradigms such as Noun-Verb association would be most useful for pre-operative language mapping [29]. Validation of word generation was confirmed by several studies which reported the sensitivity of tasks in comparison to electrically stimulated cortical mapping [33, 34].

6.3 Rhyming

This task is used for determining two visually presented rhyming words [32]. Rhyming also activates the dominant Broca's area stronger than Wernicke's area and is more specific for determining the laterality index value than word generation [35]. Mark et al. (2021) used rhyming as a relevant clinical fMRI language task to compare the language area activation pattern in multi-band gradient echo sequence with conventional fMRI sequence (Fig. 3) [36].

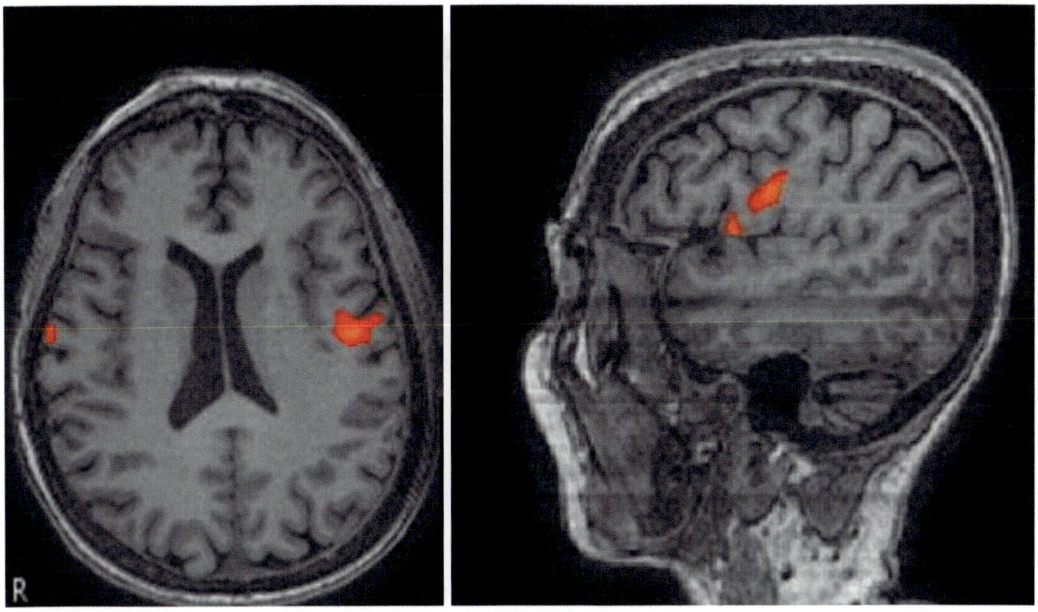

Fig. 2 The result of silent word generation task in a 27 year-old right-handed patient with epilepsy. Activation area was seen dominantly in the left IFG

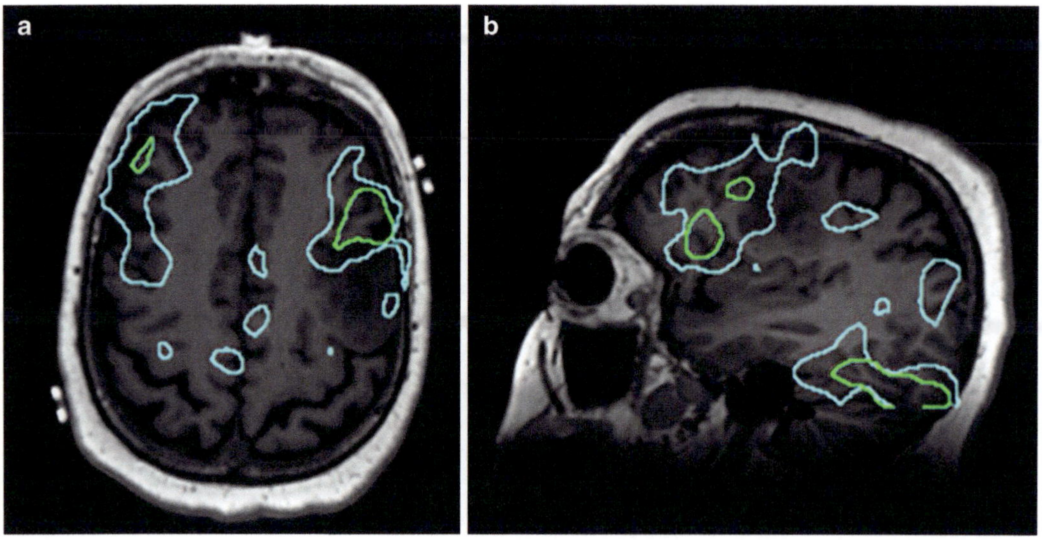

Fig. 3 Rhyming tasks performed in a 61-year-old female with a left frontal low-grade glioma. (**a**) and (**b**) are axial and sagittal images showing more widespread and robust activation during the rhyming task with the multiband sequence (cyan, acceleration factor = 6, TR 333 ms) than the traditional sequence (green, TR 2000 ms) when employing the same statistical threshold ($t = 2.5$) (License Number: 5466070696670) [36]

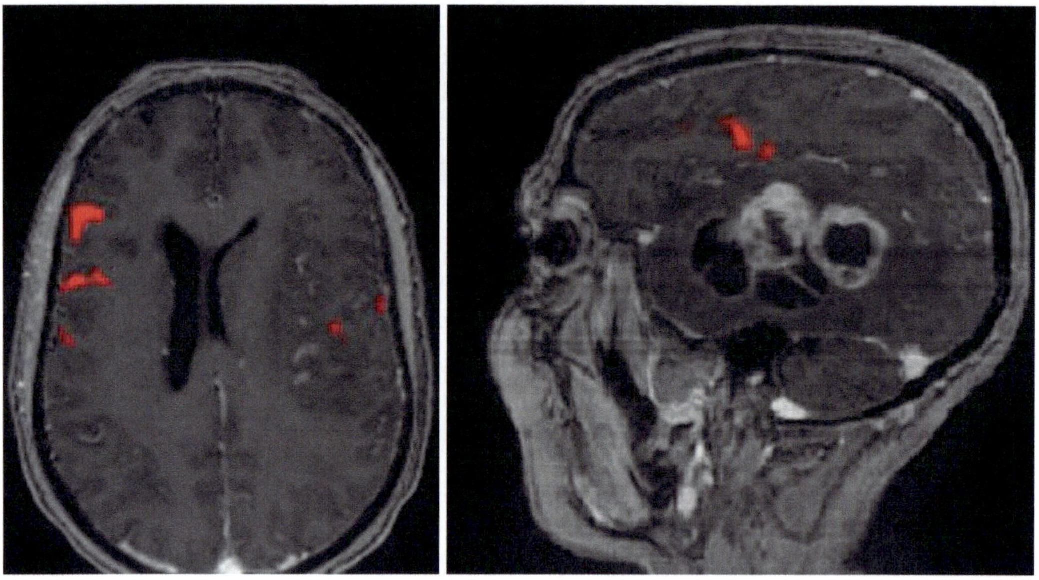

Fig. 4 Active regions during object naming task in 55 years old, right-handed female patient with left temporal-insular-frontal high-grade glioma

6.4 Object Naming

When this visual task is presented, the patient should name objects represented on the screen silently [37]. This task is used to assess semantic and lexical retrieval, and therefore activation in the frontal, parietal, and temporal lobes are expected. Because this task is easy to perform especially in patients with cognitive impairment or illiteracy, clinical assessment is often utilized frequently during awake surgery. Figure 4 shows

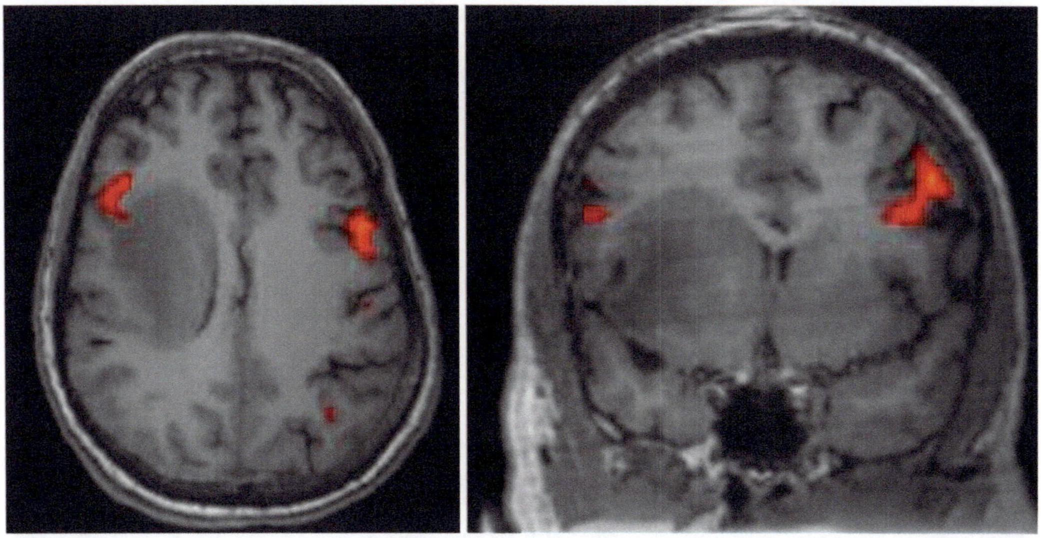

Fig. 5 Active regions during action naming task in 51 years old, right-handed, female patient with right insular low-grade glioma

axial and sagittal views in a subject with high-grade cystic glioma after performing an object naming task. Activation areas in both frontal regions were preserved as requested by the neurosurgeon and other regions were removed. Notably, for language areas related to the temporal lobe, another comprehension task was applied.

6.5 Auditory Responsive Naming

The description of an object aurally was presented and then the patient was asked to silently name the object described. This task activated the temporal lobe, with more distribution in the dominant anterior temporal region. Posterior temporal also showed activation during responsive naming task [38].

6.6 Action Naming

When this visual task is presented, the patient is asked to name the third-person singular verb form of action shown on the screen. As verb processing takes place in a separate noun region, this task might be useful for detecting the critical left prefrontal cortex and IFG (Fig. 5), where it is involved in verb processing [39, 40].

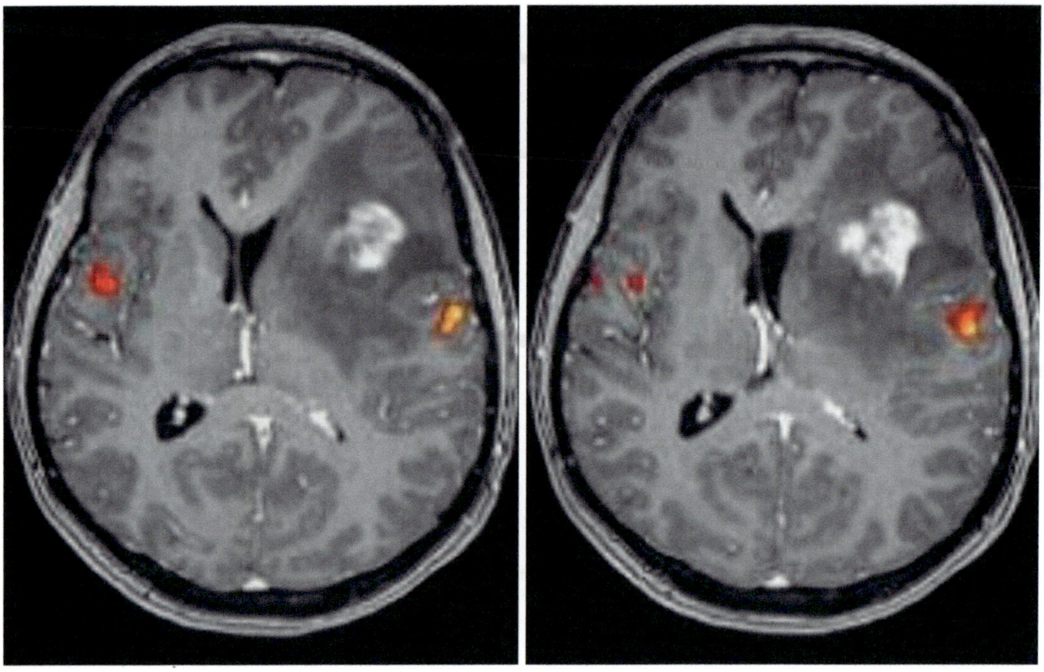

Fig. 6 Activation areas for RWR task in a right-handed patient with high-grade glioma. IFG was activated dominantly in the left side

6.7 Reverse Word Reading (RWR)

A visual task was presented, and while the letters were being shown in the reverse order, the patient was asked to read the word silently (e.g., eivom is reverse order to movie) [41]. RWR is a phonologic and orthographic task which activates classical Broca (Fig. 6) and the posterior language areas [30].

6.8 Passive Story Listening Task

To map the receptive language area, comprehension tasks are used like semantic judgment, listening to a story, or reading written language [42]. Figure 7 is a sample illustration for presurgical planning before awake craniotomy in a patient with low-grade glioma in the left posterior superior temporal lobe. Story listening task was run for the patient to examine the receptive

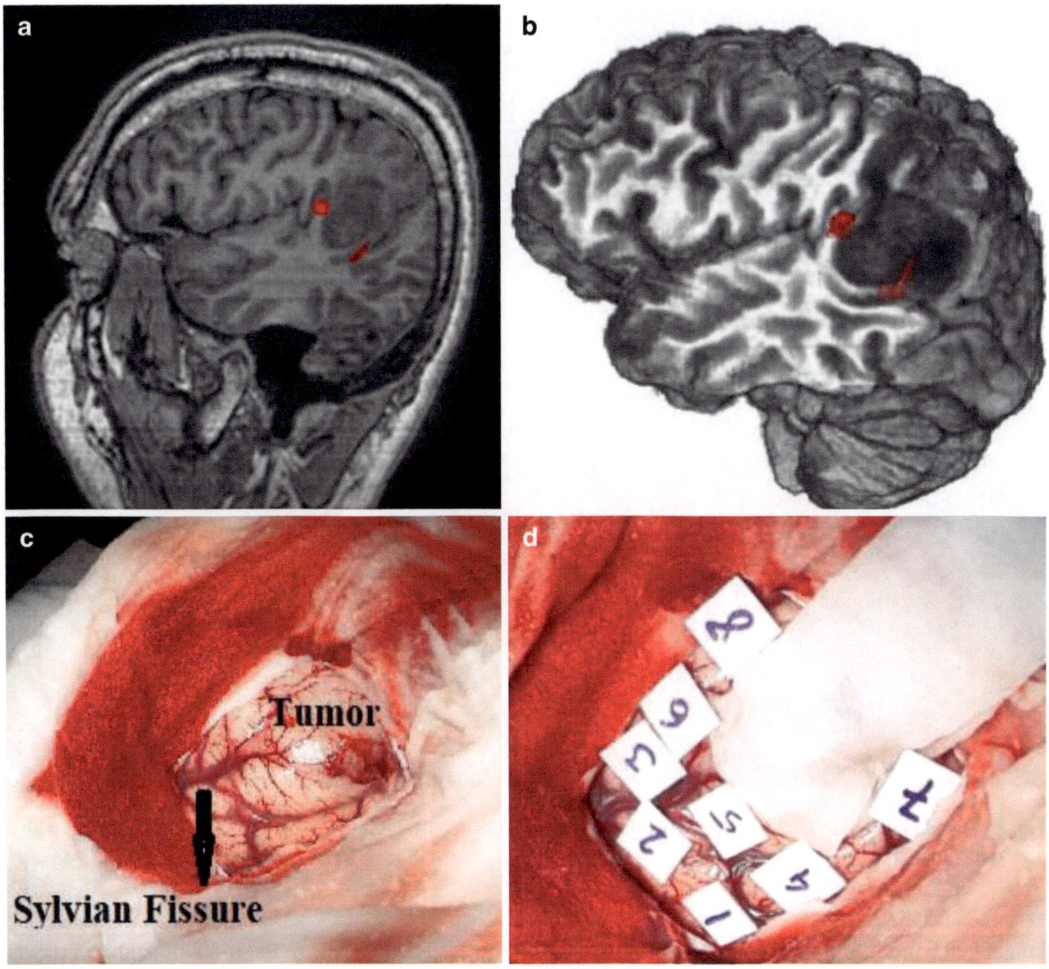

Fig. 7 (**a**) Activation area during story listening task in a patient with posterior temporal low-grade glioma. (**b**) 3D reconstruction of activation using homemade software [43]. (**c**) opening site for surgery, the location of tumor and sylvian fissure is marked. (**d**) the numbering was designed for awake cortical mapping (for more details read Sect. 6.8)

language area, as can be seen by two activation areas, one anterior of the tumor, and the other inferior to the tumor were analyzed. Interestingly, the stimulation of regions number 4 and 7 (Fig. 7d) caused language arrest during a word reading task.

7 Resting-State fMRI (rs-fMRI)

Task fMRI is commonly used for pre-surgical evaluation of motor and language networks. Although this method is very effective to identify eloquent regions within the brain in association with given tasks, rs-fMRI is an alternative form to find brain functional networks. Biswal and colleagues (1995) were pioneer researchers that suggested the utilization of intrinsic brain activity for functional localization. They demonstrated that the BOLD signal in the resting state is correlated with the somatomotor system [44]. This finding supports the possibility for future clinical application in pre-surgical planning [45–49]. Using rs-fMRI is simpler and there is no need for task presentation devices such as visual or auditory tools. If fMRI is not possible because of aphasia,

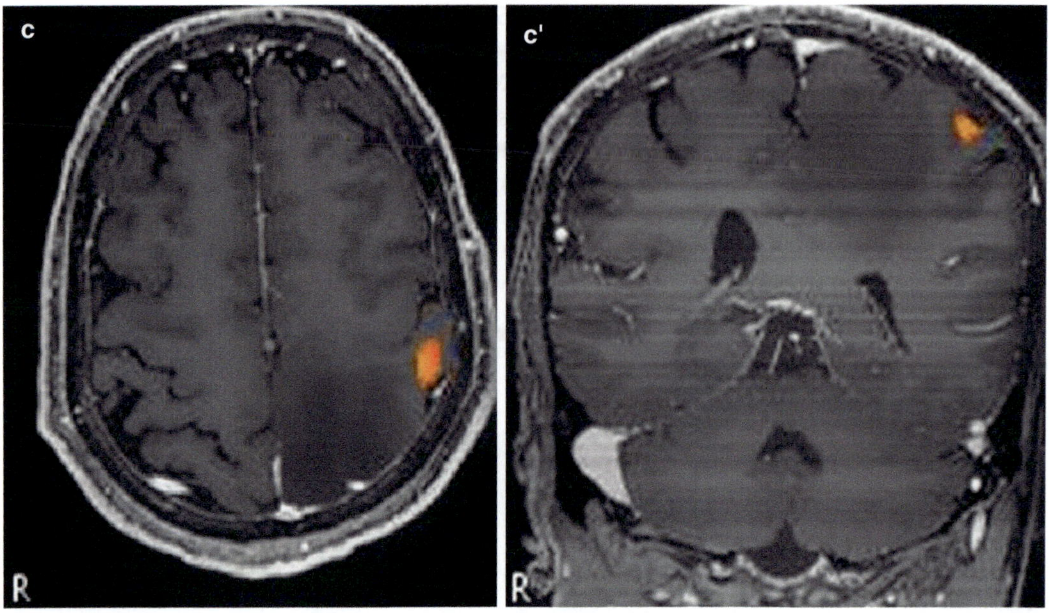

Fig. 9 (continued)

(Fig. 9b). For lesions with parasagittal involvement, we ran the foot motor task by asking the patients to move foot fingers. The foot motor area was seen after data analysis (Fig. 9a). Localization of somatosensory area for hand was performed by putting a rough plate under the hand and the patient was asked to rub the plate. However, this form of sensory function, resulted in indirect activation of pre-central gyrus, which was distinguishable in the analysis procedure by using local masks to eliminate the motor area (Fig. 9c). In other institutions, the automatic tactile stimulation used for sensory area detection led to activation only in somatosensory cortex [54].

When hand motor task is difficult for a patient to apply, due to lesion pressure, hemiparesis, or sedation, the passive movement should be performed by another person. Even if the patient imagines the hand movement, it could change the BOLD signal in contralateral pre-central hand area.

For the lip task, the patient was asked to move the lips by mimicking kissing and laughing-like motion. For tongue task, the patient was asked to move the tongue up and down (Fig. 10).

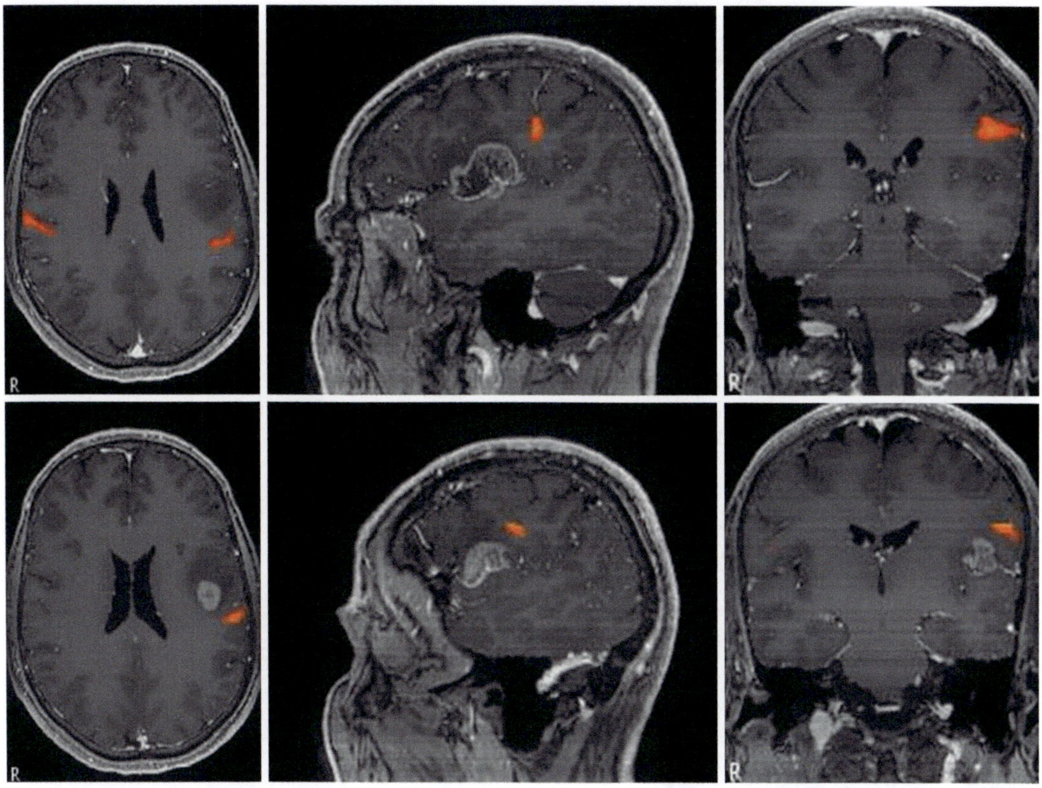

Fig. 10 performed fMRI with lip and tongue tasks for 51 years old right-handed male with a high-grade glioma in the left temporal insular frontal lobe. Upper row shows the lip motor area activation. Lower row shows the tongue motor area activation

10 Diffusion Tensor Imaging

Human brain connections have been studied by many functional and structural techniques. Fiber tracking or tractography is one of those methods which can directly probe the brain white matter, structural connectivity, and even neurite orientation. fMRI measures changes in the BOLD signal and DTI as a natural extension of diffusion imaging and estimates white matter tract directionality. Anisotropic water diffusion within the axonal fibers was calculated on the basis of high diffusion parallel to axon direction and restricted diffusion in the perpendicular direction. Diffusion tensor was calculated along six or more gradients and represented the directionality of fiber tracts, to map the directionality. Scalar mapping such as fractional anisotropy (FA) can be visualized from tensor and color-coded FA used to represent the orientation of fibers. DTI provides information about tract orientation, displacement, and disruption in case of brain tumors. Language and motor pathways are of interest for presurgical mapping.

10.1 Language Network

For lesions located in the perisylvian regions, insula, posterior aspect of inferior frontal, temporal and parietal lobe, and the adjacent white matter, language network is required. The most critical and modern language network consists of dorsal and ventral streams.

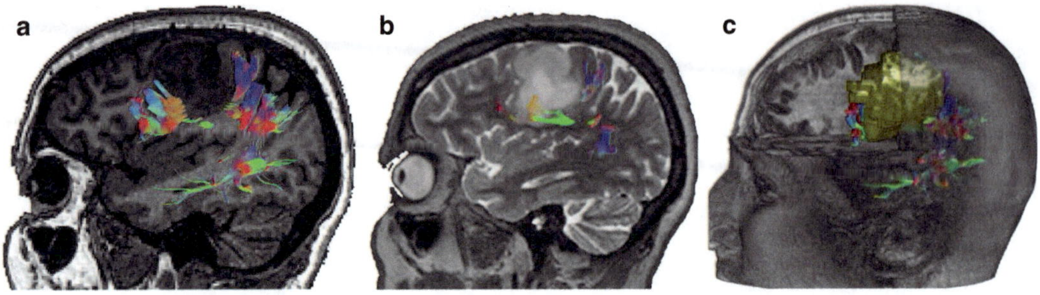

Fig. 11 SLF was segmented using ExploreDTI software [55] for 60 years old right-handed woman with a large low-grade glioma in the left frontal lobe. 2D sagittal section of T1-weighted image which overlaid by 3D SLF (**a**). Sagittal T2-weighted image overlaid with SLF shows the involvement of the tract in the corresponding section, part of SLFII is seen inside the tumor (**b**). 3D reconstruction of the data shows that the SLFII is invaded by the tumor (**c**). (**b** and **c**) were provided using homemade software [43]

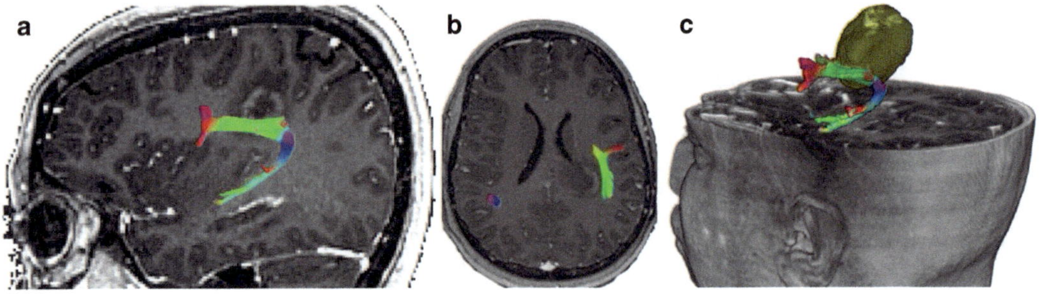

Fig. 12 AF was segmented using ExploreDTI software for 19 years old left-handed woman with a medium size high-grade glioma in the left frontal lobe. 2D sagittal section of post-contrast T1-weighted image which overlaid by 3D AF (**a**). Axial post-contrast T1-weighted image overlaid with AF shows the tumor distance to tract in the corresponding section, anterior part of AF is seen close to the tumor (**b**). 3D reconstruction of the data shows the proximity of AF and tumor (**c**)

10.1.1 Dorsal Pathway

Superior longitudinal fasciculus (SLF) and its sub-components (Fig. 11) are the important tracts in language and speech processing. SLF fibers originate from the temporal, occipital, and parietal then run above the insula and terminate in the frontal cortex. There were four sub-components for this bundle, which were described first by Petrides and Pandya [56] using autoradiography provided the divisions of SLF I, II, III, and the IV component or AF. The dorsal component, SLF I, originates from the medial and dorsal parietal, and projects ventrally along the cingulate gyrus and terminates in the dorsal and medial portion of the frontal cortex (PMA and SMA). SLF I is not involved mainly in language process, as it plays a role in attention and working memory [57], proprioception, and movement [58]. SLF II is derived from the angular gyrus and terminates within the dorsolateral frontal lobe (dorsal premotor). This bundle is involved in visuospatial awareness [59], visuomotor processing [60], and working memory [61]. Since SLF II ends in Exner's area, any disruption in the associated handwriting area may lead to agraphia [62]. SLF III or anterior AF originates from the supramarginal gyrus and terminates in the ventral premotor. Stimulation of that causes dysarthria and impairments in phonological and articulatory processing of language.

10.1.2 Arcuate Fasciculus (AF)

The traditional pathway of language, described as SLF IV, communicates with the receptive language area, posterior portion of the superior, middle temporal gyrus, and expressive language area, premotor, and middle frontal gyrus (Fig. 12). AF plays a major role in phonological processing [61], and its stimulation during awake surgery induces phonological disorder [63]. This pathway includes the anterior and posterior segments. Anterior AF connects the inferior parietal lobule with the IFG, and the posterior segment connects the inferior parietal lobule to the superior temporal gyrus [64]. AF has a role in verbal fluency [65] and verbal working memory [66].

10.1.3 Inferior Longitudinal Fasciculus (ILF)

This tract connects the occipital lobe to the anterior temporal lobe (Fig. 13) and is involved in several aspects of visual input processing, such as face recognition, reading, visual perception, and memory. However, patients with anterior temporal lobectomy, have not shown major deficit in relation to this bundle [67]. Stimulation of the ILF results in contralateral visual hemiagnosia which supports the role of this bundle in visual recognition.

10.1.4 Inferior Frontal Occipital Fasciculus (IFOF)

The association of this fascicle starts in the basal temporal, occipital, and parietal lobe then passes through below the insula and ends in the IFG and DLPFC (Fig. 14). Exact function of this tract is unknown, but based on some research, it probably plays a role in object recognition and linking the object to lexical labels [64]. Stimulation of this bundle in the dominant hemisphere elicited semantic paraphasia during the task of naming [68].

10.1.5 Uncinate Fasciculus (UF)

This bundle appears similar to a hook and runs between inferior frontal and anterior temporal lobe (Fig. 15). The frontal arm of UF projects

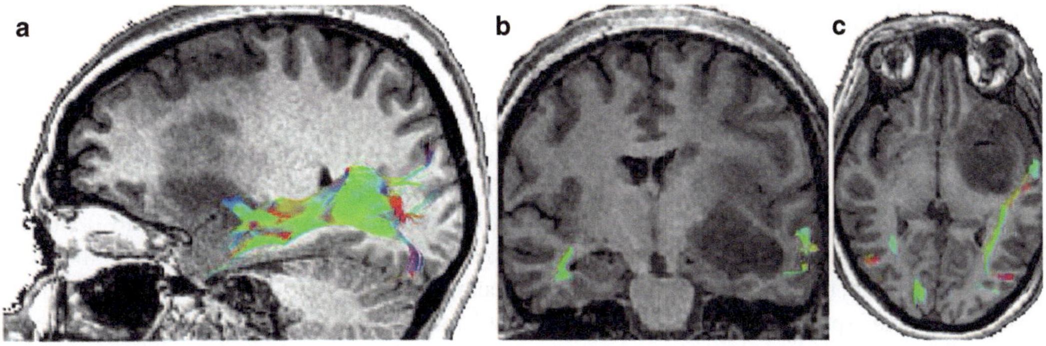

Fig. 13 ILF in 29 years old right-handed woman with a large low-grade glioma in temporal-insular-frontal lobes. Sagittal section overlaid with 3D segmented ILF (**a**). Coronal section and the ILF trajectory around the tumor in contrast to the contralateral (**b**). Axial section at the level of ILF pathway shows that the tumor pressure led to lateral displacement of the tract (**c**)

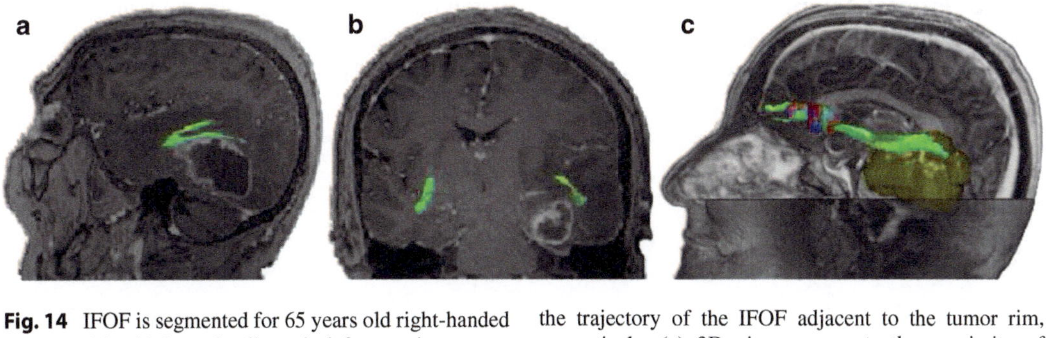

Fig. 14 IFOF is segmented for 65 years old right-handed woman with a high-grade glioma in left posterior temporal. (**a** and **b**) show the sagittal and coronal sections and the trajectory of the IFOF adjacent to the tumor rim, respectively. (**c**) 3D view represents the proximity of tumor and IFOF

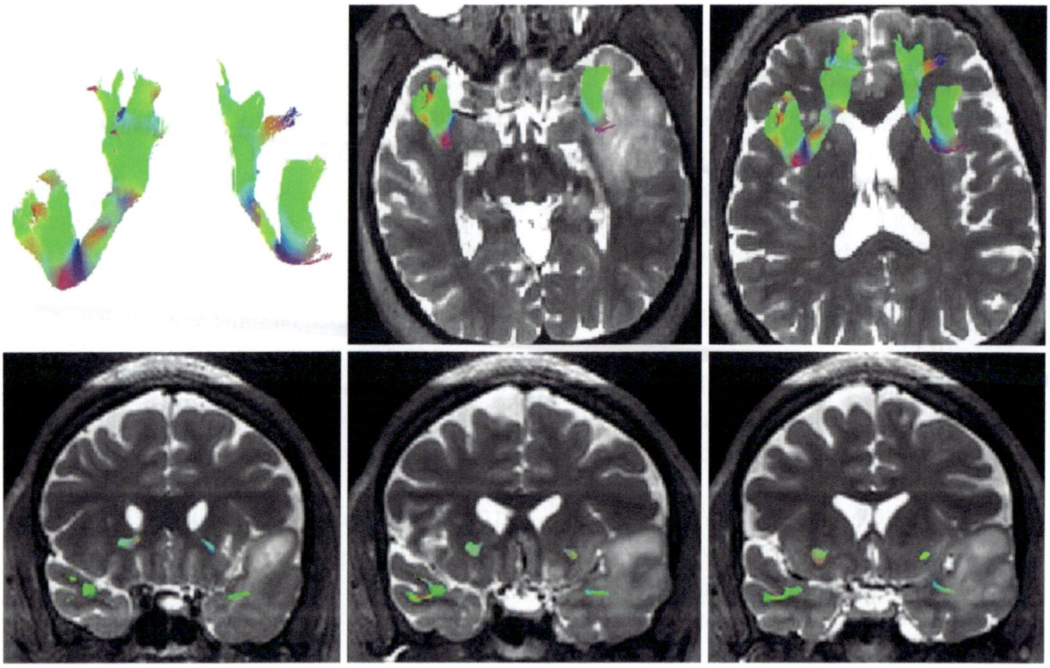

Fig. 15 Uncinate in 45 years old right-handed woman with an ill-defined tumor in left anterior temporal. Involvement of tract by edematous area and tumor is seen

into the lateral and medial orbitofrontal cortex and the temporal arm projects to the temporal pole, amygdala, anterior portion of the hippocampus, anterior parts of the superior and middle temporal gyrus. UF is a part of the limbic system and is involved in memory, emotion, semantic processing, and specific aspects of naming. Removal of UF in glioma patients results in famous face naming deficit; however, patients can retrieve biographical information about famous people [69].

10.1.6 Frontal Aslant

Frontal aslant tract is a recently studied intralobar pathway which connects Brodmann area (BA) 44 in the posterior wall of the ascending ramus of the lateral fissure (frontal opercular) to the anterior part of the SMA and pre-SMA (Fig. 16). Some fibers also project to BA 6 and because of their oblique orientation in the coronal plane, it is called aslant. The role of this tract in language processing has been reported in one patient with oligoastrocytoma grade II who experienced severe mutism after resection of tumor and deficit in adjacent aslant fibers [70]. Another study revealed that this fascicle has a role in language network by reporting the correlation between FA value of aslant and deficit in verbal fluency in patients with primary progressive aphasia [71].

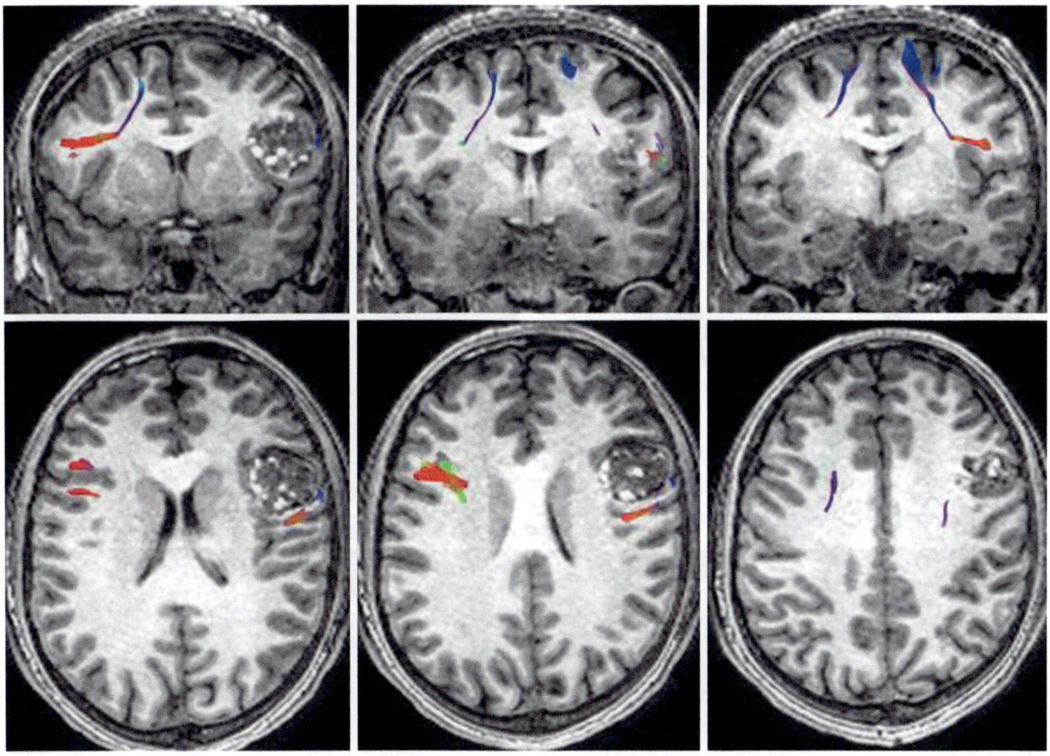

Fig. 16 Frontal Aslant in 19 years old left-handed man with an atrio-venous malformation (AVM) in left IFG. Posterolateral border of the lesion is close to the tract and mild dislocation compared to the contralateral Aslant is seen in the axial sections (lower row)

10.2 Motor Pathways

Corticospinal tract (CST) is the most eloquent pathway in the motor system which arises from the upper two-thirds of the precentral gyrus (primary motor area, M1, BA 4). Some fibers from postcentral gyrus (primary sensory cortex, BA 1, 2, and 3) contribute to this pathway. One-third of the CST is formed from SMA and premotor fibers. These projecting fibers in the M1 have somatotopic organization such as the leg and foot fibers which are located in dorsal and medial aspects of M1; the hand area is located in lateral aspect; and the face and tongue fibers arise from ventral and inferior of M1. After leaving the cortex, the CST bends forward to reach the posterior limb of internal capsule. Following this pathway, the face and tongue fibers run anteriorly, and the foot and leg fibers run posteriorly. CST then passes through the cerebral peduncle and brain stem toward the anterior portion of spinal cord (Fig. 17). During electrical stimulation of CST in awake surgery, when the patient is frequently asked to move his/her extremities the result becomes problematic in regard to motor initiation and control which can range from complete arrest of movement to involuntary accelerated movement [72].

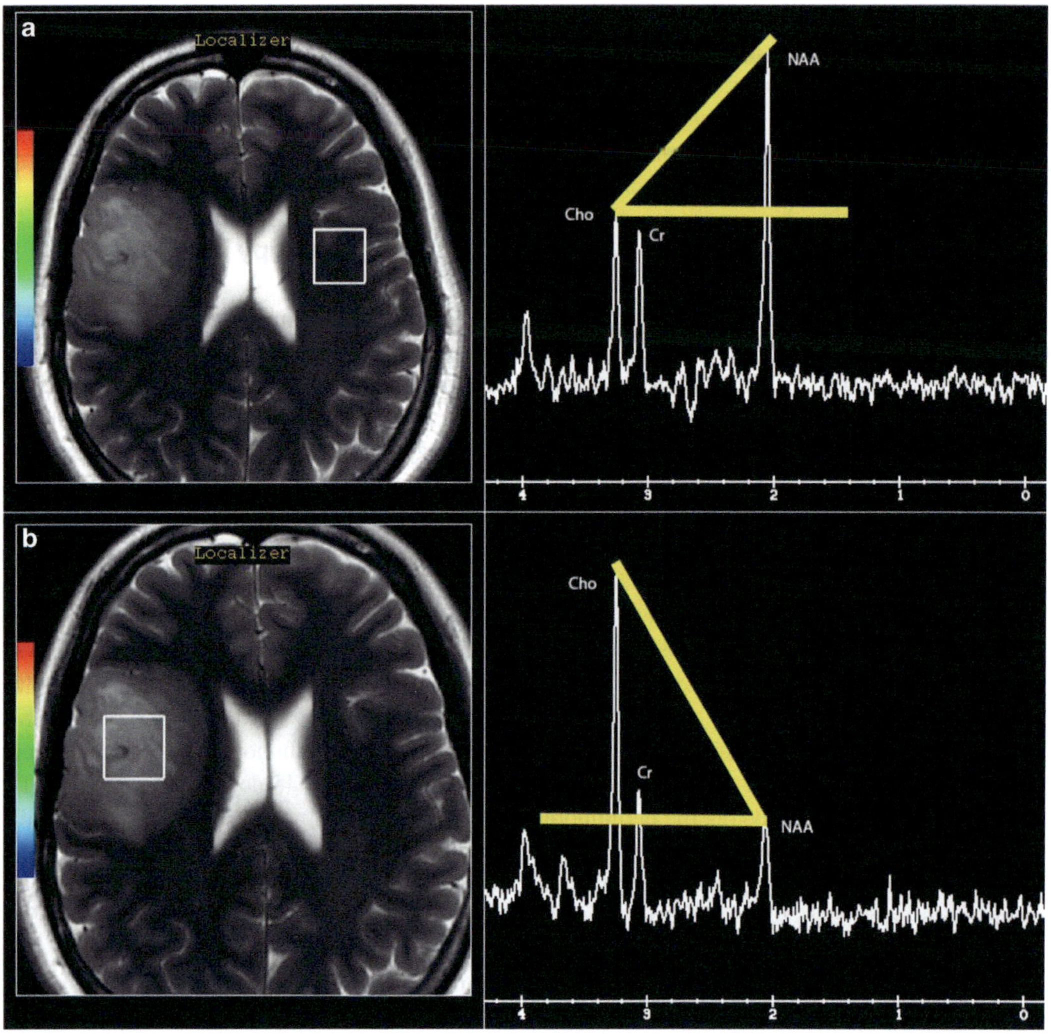

Fig. 18 (**a**) Hunter's angle in normal spectrum arrived from normal brain parenchyma. (**b**) Hunter's angle in pathologic region spectrum

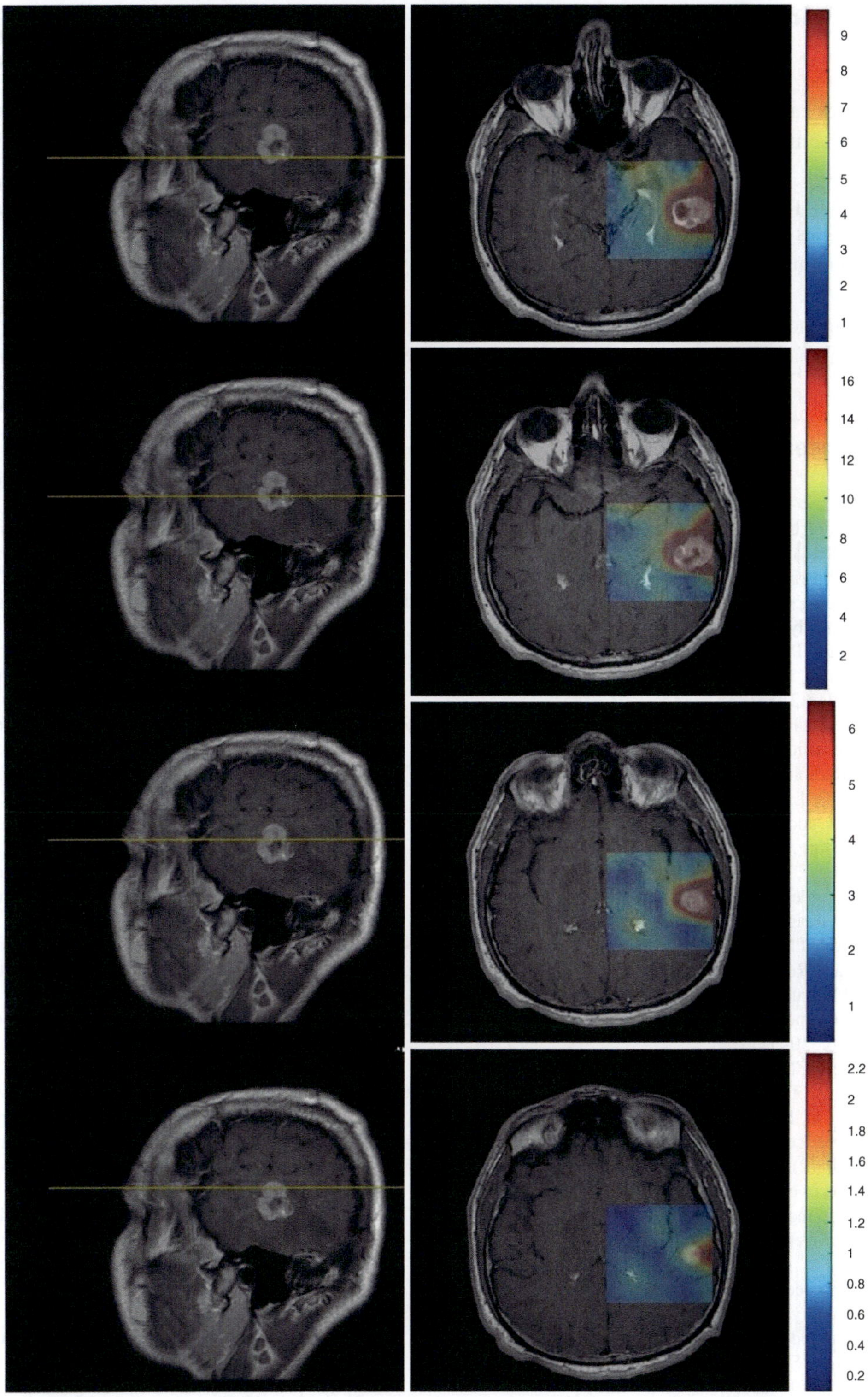

Fig. 19 Metabolic map with threshold of Cho/NAA > 1.8 which is correspond to tumor cell presence is provided using 3D MRS imaging (MRSI) in a patient with glioblastoma in the left temporal. The red color territory shows that the tumor cell invasion is greater than enhancing portion of the tumor

13 Conclusion

Despite the fact that conventional MRI and its modalities can display many lesions besides anatomic structures of the cerebrum, it is limited in determining different pathologies in the brain. With future progress toward a high-tech era, new technologies such as advanced neuroimaging have been introduced covering conventional MRI weaknesses. fMRI, DTI, MRS, and others are becoming more prominent in daily practice while improving patient outcome.

References

1. Villanueva-Meyer JE, Mabray MC, Cha S. Current clinical brain tumor imaging. Neurosurgery. 2017;81(3):397–415.
2. Scott J, Brasher P, Sevick R, et al. How often are non-enhancing supratentorial gliomas malignant? A population study. Neurology. 2002;59(6):947–9.
3. Schaefer PW, Grant PE, Gonzalez RG. Diffusion-weighted MR imaging of the brain. Radiology. 2000;217(2):331–45.
4. Yamasaki F, Kurisu K, Satoh K, et al. Apparent diffusion coefficient of human brain tumors at MR imaging. Radiology. 2005;235(3):985–91.
5. Kahn E, Lane M, Sagher O. Eloquent: history of a word's adoption into the neurosurgical lexicon. J Neurosurg. 2017;127(6):1461–6.
6. Chang EF, Clark A, Smith JS, et al. Functional mapping–guided resection of low-grade gliomas in eloquent areas of the brain: improvement of long-term survival. J Neurosurg. 2011;114(3):566–73.
7. Broca P. Remarks on the seat of the faculty of articulated language, following an observation of aphemia (loss of speech). Bulletin de la Société Anatomique. 1861;6:330–57.
8. Vanacôr CN, Isolan GR, Yu YH, et al. Microsurgical anatomy of language. Clin Anat. 2021;34(1):154–68.
9. Catani M, Dell'Acqua F, Vergani F, et al. Short frontal lobe connections of the human brain. Cortex. 2012;48(2):273–91.
10. Bookheimer S. Pre-surgical language mapping with functional magnetic resonance imaging. Neuropsychol Rev. 2007;17(2):145–55.
11. Wernicke C. The symptom complex of aphasia. In: Proceedings of the Boston Colloquium for the Philosophy of Science 1966/1968. Springer; 1969.
12. Geschwind N. Disconnexion syndromes in animals and man. Selected papers on language and the brain; 1974. p. 105–236.
13. Tremblay P, Dick AS. Broca and Wernicke are dead, or moving past the classic model of language neurobiology. Brain Lang. 2016;162:60–71.
14. Nasios G, Dardiotis E, Messinis L. From Broca and Wernicke to the neuromodulation era: insights of brain language networks for neurorehabilitation. Behav Neurol. 2019;2019:9894571.
15. Saur D, Kreher BW, Schnell S, et al. Ventral and dorsal pathways for language. Proc Natl Acad Sci. 2008;105(46):18035–40.
16. Gelfand JR, Bookheimer SY. Dissociating neural mechanisms of temporal sequencing and processing phonemes. Neuron. 2003;38(5):831–42.
17. Li Q, Ferraro GD, Pasquini L, et al. Core language brain network for fMRI language task used in clinical applications. Network Neurosci. 2020;4(1):134–54.
18. Vassal M, Le Bars E, Moritz-Gasser SS, et al. Crossed aphasia elicited by intraoperative cortical and subcortical stimulation in awake patients. J Neurosurg. 2010;113(6):1251–8.
19. Rotta JM, de Oliveira MF. Fundamentals of brain tumor surgery in eloquent areas. Arquivos Brasileiros de Neurocirurgia. 2015;34(2):122–7.
20. Sharan A, Ooi YC, Langfitt J, et al. Intracarotid amobarbital procedure for epilepsy surgery. Epilepsy Behav. 2011;20(2):209–13.
21. Sarubbo S, Tate M, De Benedictis A, et al. Mapping critical cortical hubs and white matter pathways by direct electrical stimulation: an original functional atlas of the human brain. Neuroimage. 2020;205:116237.
22. Whitney C, Kirk M, O'Sullivan J, et al. The neural organization of semantic control: TMS evidence for a distributed network in left inferior frontal and posterior middle temporal gyrus. Cereb Cortex. 2011;21(5):1066–75.
23. Bookheimer S. Functional MRI of language: new approaches to understanding the cortical organization of semantic processing. Annu Rev Neurosci. 2002;25(1):151–88.
24. Engström M, Ragnehed M, Lundberg P, et al. Paradigm design of sensory–motor and language tests in clinical fMRI. Neurophysiol Clin. 2004;34(6):267–77.
25. Chee MW, O'Craven KM, Bergida R, et al. Auditory and visual word processing studied with fMRI. Hum Brain Mapp. 1999;7(1):15–28.
26. Zacà D, Nickerson JP, Deib G, et al. Effectiveness of four different clinical fMRI paradigms for preoperative regional determination of language lateralization in patients with brain tumors. Neuroradiology. 2012;54(9):1015–25.
27. Ischebeck A, Indefrey P, Usui N, et al. Reading in a regular orthography: an FMRI study investigating the role of visual familiarity. J Cogn Neurosci. 2004;16(5):727–41.
28. El Salek K, Hassan IS, Kotrotsou A, et al. Silent sentence completion shows superiority localizing Wernicke's area and activation patterns of distinct language paradigms correlate with genomics: prospective study. Sci Rep. 2017;7(1):1–8.
29. Zaca D, Jarso S, Pillai JJ. Role of semantic paradigms for optimization of language mapping in clinical FMRI studies. Am J Neuroradiol. 2013;34(10):1966–71.

30. Mahdavi A, Houshmand S, Oghabian MA, et al. Developing optimized fMRI protocol for clinical use: comparison of different language paradigms. J Magn Reson Imaging. 2011;34(2):413–9.
31. Lehericy S, Cohen L, Bazin B, et al. Functional MR evaluation of temporal and frontal language dominance compared with the Wada test. Neurology. 2000;54(8):1625–33.
32. Lurito JT, Kareken DA, Lowe MJ, et al. Comparison of rhyming and word generation with FMRI. Hum Brain Mapp. 2000;10(3):99–106.
33. Yetkin FZ, Mueller WM, Morris GL, et al. Functional MR activation correlated with intraoperative cortical mapping. Am J Neuroradiol. 1997;18(7):1311–5.
34. Brannen JH, Badie B, Moritz CH, et al. Reliability of functional MR imaging with word-generation tasks for mapping Broca's area. Am J Neuroradiol. 2001;22(9):1711–8.
35. Pillai JJ, Zaca D. Relative utility for hemispheric lateralization of different clinical fMRI activation tasks within a comprehensive language paradigm battery in brain tumor patients as assessed by both threshold-dependent and threshold-independent analysis methods. Neuroimage. 2011;54:S136–45.
36. Mark IT, Black DF, DeLone DR, et al. Higher temporal resolution multiband fMRI provides improved presurgical language maps. Neuroradiology. 2021;63(3):439–45.
37. Benson R, FitzGerald D, LeSueur L, et al. Language dominance determined by whole brain functional MRI in patients with brain lesions. Neurology. 1999;52(4):798.
38. Farias ST, Harrington G, Broomand C, et al. Differences in functional MR imaging activation patterns associated with confrontation naming and responsive naming. Am J Neuroradiol. 2005;26(10):2492–9.
39. Pillon A, d'Honincthun P. The organization of the conceptual system: the case of the "object versus action" dimension. Cogn Neuropsychol. 2010;27(7):587–613.
40. Rofes A, Miceli G. Language mapping with verbs and sentences in awake surgery: a review. Neuropsychol Rev. 2014;24(2):185–99.
41. Mahdavi A, Azar R, Shoar MH, et al. Functional MRI in clinical practice: assessment of language and motor for pre-surgical planning. Neuroradiol J. 2015;28(5):468–73.
42. Sunaert S. Presurgical planning for tumor resectioning. J Magn Reson Imaging. 2006;23(6):887–905.
43. Shakeri M. Smart Assistant Surgeon (Onyx). Bita Negar Afzar. 2017. https://binasoft.ir/.
44. Biswal B, Zerrin Yetkin F, Haughton VM, et al. Functional connectivity in the motor cortex of resting human brain using echo-planar MRI. Magn Reson Med. 1995;34(4):537–41.
45. Tie Y, Rigolo L, Norton IH, et al. Defining language networks from resting-state fMRI for surgical planning—a feasibility study. Hum Brain Mapp. 2014;35(3):1018–30.
46. Branco P, Seixas D, Deprez S, et al. Resting-state functional magnetic resonance imaging for language preoperative planning. Front Hum Neurosci. 2016;10:11.
47. Park KY, Lee JJ, Dierker D, et al. Mapping language function with task-based vs. resting-state functional MRI. PloS One. 2020;15(7):e0236423.
48. Zhang D, Johnston JM, Fox MD, et al. Preoperative sensorimotor mapping in brain tumor patients using spontaneous fluctuations in neuronal activity imaged with functional magnetic resonance imaging: initial experience. Neurosurgery. 2009;65(Suppl_6):226–36.
49. Yahyavi-Firouz-Abadi N, Pillai J, Lindquist M, et al. Presurgical brain mapping of the ventral somatomotor network in patients with brain tumors using resting-state fMRI. Am J Neuroradiol. 2017;38(5):1006–12.
50. Chouinard PA, Paus T. The primary motor and premotor areas of the human cerebral cortex. Neuroscientist. 2006;12(2):143–52.
51. Hill VB, Cankurtaran CZ, Liu BP, et al. A practical review of functional MRI anatomy of the language and motor systems. Am J Neuroradiol. 2019;40(7):1084–90.
52. Nachev P, Wydell H, O'neill K, et al. The role of the pre-supplementary motor area in the control of action. Neuroimage. 2007;36:T155–63.
53. Alario F-X, Chainay H, Lehericy S, et al. The role of the supplementary motor area (SMA) in word production. Brain Res. 2006;1076(1):129–43.
54. Stippich C, Romanowski A, Nennig E, et al. Fully automated localization of the human primary somatosensory cortex in one minute by functional magnetic resonance imaging. Neurosci Lett. 2004;364(2):90–3.
55. Leemans A, Jeurissen B, Sijbers J, et al. ExploreDTI: a graphical toolbox for processing, analyzing, and visualizing diffusion MR data. In: Proceedings of the International Society for Magnetic Resonance in Medicine; 2009.
56. Petrides M, Pandya DN. Projections to the frontal cortex from the posterior parietal region in the rhesus monkey. J Comp Neurol. 1984;228(1):105–16.
57. Nakajima R, Kinoshita M, Shinohara H, et al. The superior longitudinal fascicle: reconsidering the fronto-parietal neural network based on anatomy and function. Brain Imaging Behav. 2020;14(6):2817–30.
58. Chang EF, Raygor KP, Berger MS. Contemporary model of language organization: an overview for neurosurgeons. J Neurosurg. 2015;122(2):250–61.
59. Nakajima R, Kinoshita M, Miyashita K, et al. Damage of the right dorsal superior longitudinal fascicle by awake surgery for glioma causes persistent visuospatial dysfunction. Sci Rep. 2017;7(1):1–10.
60. Budisavljevic S, Dell'Acqua F, Zanatto D, et al. Asymmetry and structure of the fronto-parietal networks underlie visuomotor processing in humans. Cereb Cortex. 2017;27(2):1532–44.
61. Duffau H, Moritz-Gasser S, Mandonnet E. A re-examination of neural basis of language processing: proposal of a dynamic hodotopical model from data

provided by brain stimulation mapping during picture naming. Brain Lang. 2014;131:1–10.
62. Klein E, Willmes K, Jung S, et al. Differing connectivity of Exner's area for numbers and letters. Front Hum Neurosci. 2016;10:281.
63. Sarubbo S, De Benedictis A, Merler S, et al. Towards a functional atlas of human white matter. Hum Brain Mapp. 2015;36(8):3117–36.
64. Catani M, Mesulam M. The arcuate fasciculus and the disconnection theme in language and aphasia: history and current state. Cortex. 2008;44(8):953–61.
65. Li M, Zhang Y, Song L, et al. Structural connectivity subserving verbal fluency revealed by lesion-behavior mapping in stroke patients. Neuropsychologia. 2017;101:85–96.
66. Meyer L, Cunitz K, Obleser J, et al. Sentence processing and verbal working memory in a white-matter-disconnection patient. Neuropsychologia. 2014;61:190–6.
67. Ramos-Fresnedo A, Segura-Duran I, Chaichana KL, et al. Supratentorial white matter tracts. In: Comprehensive overview of modern surgical approaches to intrinsic brain tumors. Amsterdam: Elsevier; 2019. p. 23–35.
68. Duffau H, Gatignol P, Mandonnet E, et al. Intraoperative subcortical stimulation mapping of language pathways in a consecutive series of 115 patients with Grade II glioma in the left dominant hemisphere. J Neurosurg. 2008;109(3):461–71.
69. Papagno C, Miracapillo C, Casarotti A, et al. What is the role of the uncinate fasciculus? Surgical removal and proper name retrieval. Brain. 2011;134(2):405–14.
70. Bizzi A. Diffusion imaging with MR tractography for brain tumor surgery. In: Clinical functional MRI. New York: Springer; 2022. p. 249–314.
71. Catani M, Mesulam MM, Jakobsen E, et al. A novel frontal pathway underlies verbal fluency in primary progressive aphasia. Brain. 2013;136(8):2619–28.
72. Schucht P, Moritz-Gasser S, Herbet G, et al. Subcortical electrostimulation to identify network subserving motor control. Hum Brain Mapp. 2013;34(11):3023–30.
73. Provenzale JM, Mukundan S, Barboriak DP. Diffusion-weighted and perfusion MR imaging for brain tumor characterization and assessment of treatment response. Radiology. 2006;239(3):632–49.
74. Cha S, Knopp EA, Johnson G, et al. Intracranial mass lesions: dynamic contrast-enhanced susceptibility-weighted echo-planar perfusion MR imaging. Radiology. 2002;223(1):11–29.
75. Essig M, Nguyen TB, Shiroishi MS, et al. Perfusion MRI: the five most frequently asked clinical questions. AJR Am J Roentgenol. 2013;201(3):W495.
76. Law M, Yang S, Wang H, et al. Glioma grading: sensitivity, specificity, and predictive values of perfusion MR imaging and proton MR spectroscopic imaging compared with conventional MR imaging. Am J Neuroradiol. 2003;24(10):1989–98.
77. Belkić D, Belkić K. A meta-analysis of studies using MR spectroscopy for evaluating suspicious lesions after radiation therapy of primary brain tumors. J Math Chem. 2012;50(9):2527–57.
78. Lin A, Ross BD, Harris K, et al. Efficacy of proton magnetic resonance spectroscopy in neurological diagnosis and neurotherapeutic decision making. NeuroRx. 2005;2(2):197–214.
79. Julià-Sapé M, Coronel I, Majós C, et al. Prospective diagnostic performance evaluation of single-voxel 1H MRS for typing and grading of brain tumours. NMR Biomed. 2012;25(4):661–73.
80. McIntyre DJ, Madhu B, Lee S-H, et al. Magnetic resonance spectroscopy of cancer metabolism and response to therapy. Radiat Res. 2012;177(4):398–435.
81. Majós C, Bruna J, Julia-Sape M, et al. Proton MR spectroscopy provides relevant prognostic information in high-grade astrocytomas. Am J Neuroradiol. 2011;32(1):74–80.
82. Parra NA, Maudsley AA, Gupta RK, et al. Volumetric spectroscopic imaging of glioblastoma multiforme radiation treatment volumes. Int J Radiat Oncol Biol Phys. 2014;90(2):376–84.
83. Ramesh K, Mellon EA, Gurbani SS, Weinberg BD, Schreibmann E, Sheriff SA, Goryawala M, De Le Fuente M, Eaton BR, Zhong J, Voloschin AD. A multi-institutional pilot clinical trial of spectroscopic MRI-guided radiation dose escalation for newly diagnosed glioblastoma. Neuro-oncology advances. 2022;4(1):vdac006
84. Raminfard S, Haghighatkhah H, Alimohamadi M, et al. Assessment of residual tumor after resection of glioma: a magnetic resonance spectroscopic study. Arch Neurosci 2019;6(Brain Mapping).
85. Pirzkall A, Li X, Oh J, et al. 3D MRSI for resected high-grade gliomas before RT: tumor extent according to metabolic activity in relation to MRI. Int J Radiat Oncol Biol Phys. 2004;59(1):126–37.
86. Wang X, Hu X, Xie P, et al. Comparison of magnetic resonance spectroscopy and positron emission tomography in detection of tumor recurrence in posttreatment of glioma: a diagnostic meta-analysis. Asia Pac J Clin Oncol. 2015;11(2):97–105.
87. Stadlbauer A, Moser E, Gruber S, et al. Improved delineation of brain tumors: an automated method for segmentation based on pathologic changes of 1H-MRSI metabolites in gliomas. Neuroimage. 2004;23(2):454–61.
88. Ricci R, Bacci A, Tugnoli V, et al. Metabolic findings on 3T 1H-MR spectroscopy in peritumoral brain edema. Am J Neuroradiol. 2007;28(7):1287–91.
89. Zhang J, Zhuang D-X, Yao C-J, et al. Metabolic approach for tumor delineation in glioma surgery: 3D MR spectroscopy image–guided resection. J Neurosurg. 2016;124(6):1585–93.

Principles of Neuroanesthesia for Awake Craniotomy <Neuroanesthesia, Awake Craniotomy>

Reza Shariat Moharari and Gilda Barzin

1 Introduction

Craniotomy on awake patients is an important technique widely used in brain surgery for certain intracranial lesions. This technique is generally indicated for treatment of neurological conditions that require patient cooperation, and is classified into four categories: functional surgery, tumor resection, resection of vascular lesions, and minor intracranial procedures (such as ventriculostomy, stereotactic biopsy, and brain endoscopy) [1]. Functional surgery is a technique utilized in conditions which demands accurate electrographic mapping and recording of electrophysiological signals which is quite similar to epilepsy surgery as well as deep brain stimulation (DBS) and is common in Parkinson's disease. When intervention is necessary and near a part of the brain that controls vision, movement, or speech, the patient may need to be awake during surgery [2–5] so that the anesthesiologist can ask questions and monitor the activity as well as pulses in the brain.

For a successful awake craniotomy, patients should be carefully selected, briefed, and prepared by the anesthesiologist because optimal anesthesia management is crucial during the procedure. Contrary to what the phrase 'awake craniotomy' may indicate, the patient is not completely awake during the entire surgery, and the stimulating phase of the operation requires different levels of anesthesia or sedation. Nonetheless, during the mapping and tumor resection phases, the patient should be completely awake. The two anesthesia techniques used in awake craniotomy are conscious sedation and the asleep-awake ± asleep techniques [2, 6]. Analgesia may be induced through intravenous (IV) injection of analgesics, local anesthesia, or scalp block. The main objectives of this approach are maximizing patient cooperation, maintaining general hemostasis, minimizing possible interactions between anesthetic agents, and electrophysiological recordings.

In awake craniotomy, effective teamwork (i.e., neurosurgeon, neuroanesthesiologist, neuropsychiatrist, neurologist, neuroelectrophysiologist, and neuroradiologist) and close collaboration between neurosurgeons and anesthesiologists are of great importance to secure patient satisfaction through maximizing their compliance and reducing stress during the operation. Although anesthetic techniques have greatly improved, those required in awake craniotomy need further clarification, and more research is needed to expand

R. S. Moharari (✉) · G. Barzin
Department of Anesthesiology, Sina Hospital, Tehran University of Medical Sciences, Tehran, Iran
e-mail: moharari@tums.ac.ir

A. Pour-Rashidi, J. Aarabi (eds.), *The Principles of Successful Awake Craniotomy*,
https://doi.org/10.1007/978-981-99-2985-6_6

Table 2 Contraindications of awake craniotomy

Absolute contraindications	Noncompliance of the patient
	Inability to remain motionless during the operation
	Lack of cooperation
Relative contraindications	Severe or mild cough
	Difficulty in learning and cooperation
	Difficulty to lay flat
	Neurological and psychiatric problems such as severe anxiety
	Any history of psychiatric problems such as mood instability
	Cognitive disorders
	Somnolence
	Confusion
	Dysphagia
	Language barriers
	Obstructive sleep apnea
	Addiction
	Smoking
	Morbid obesity or high body mass index
	Higher American Society of Anesthesiology classification scale score
	Seizure
	Young age

tions, such as congestive heart failure with ejection fraction less than 10%; and late stages of pregnancy when there is the risk of neurological crisis [6]. Tumor characteristics such as size, pathologic features, and vascularity can also influence the surgeon's decision about choosing awake brain surgery based on their experience and potential for collaboration at their institution. More details concerning relative and absolute contraindications of awake craniotomy are tabulated in Table 2.

5 Preoperative Preparations

In order to increase the success rate of awake craniotomy surgery, there are preparatory stages (physical and psychological) which should be considered preoperatively. Initially, patients should be selected based on eligibility criteria (awake craniotomy indications) and the surgical team should brief them the day before surgery, as patient cooperation is imperative for the success of the operation and minimization of potential complications [2]. When evaluating patients, careful consideration of their past medical history and comorbidities, the rate of potential complications, and the failure of the procedure can be significantly reduced. In addition, medical examination of the patients should include a particular focus on neurological aspects that may negatively affect the surgery and its outcome. For example, seizures are a relatively common condition which may complicate the surgery during awake craniotomy with grave consequences. If a patient has a history of seizures, detailed information regarding the type of seizure, frequency, and duration should be obtained and recorded prior to the procedure [2, 21, 22].

One of the most challenging aspects of awake craniotomy is airway management. Since the operation is conducted on the scalp, it is not possible for the anesthesiologist to stand behind the patient during the procedure, so reintubation during the operation is extremely difficult. Therefore, patients with compromised airways or any history of difficult intubation or obstructive sleep apnea are poor candidates for this type of surgery and the rate of failure is considerably high.

Key factors in managing the patient's anxiety level should be evaluated preoperatively. Thorough consultation before the procedure can significantly decrease the anxiety of the patients. Patients should be briefed about the details of the awake craniotomy procedure and aware of what to expect. Environmental features (such as the operating room atmosphere, positioning, immobility, fixed head, the scalp nerve block, possible discomfort, and the motor and language test) should be clearly described either verbally or in writing. For example, patients are informed that they should not attempt to move their heads during the operation (as this might breach drape sterility and hinder brain mapping) and understand that their heads will be fixed in a Mayfield headrest. Ideally, the anesthesia consultation should not only include a brief tour of the operating room and the environment, sighting the equipment, but the auditory sounds that may occur throughout the procedure. This can play a crucial role in alleviating patient anxiety. In some centers, a few days prior to the surgery, the team (i.e., neurosurgeon, neuroanesthesiologist, neuropsychiatrist, neurologist, neuroelectrophysiologist, and neuroradiologist) practice the functional tests (speech and motor) with the patient and a baseline assessment is recorded, which is used later to compare the patient's performance during the operation. Establishment of rapport between the patient and the team can play a pivotal role in the operation's success by encouraging patient cooperation and formation of trust which is established by familiarizing them with the details of the procedure.

6 Theater Arrangement

Awake craniotomy requires effective communication between the entire operating room staff. Patients should be familiarized with the importance of constant face-to-face interaction during the surgery, positioning, immobility, head immobilization, environmental ambient noises, urinary catheter insertion, and mapping-related tasks [23]. Functional testing (i.e., motor and speech) needs to be practiced at this stage. For example, during language testing, the anesthesiologist or neuropsychologist may practice counting forwards or backwards from 1 to 10 or naming a set of pictures the day before the surgery. The motor test includes squeezing the anesthesiologist's hand or moving their hand in a waving motion. For each of these tests, written instructions should be prepared for the patients so they can review them the night before surgery.

Standard monitoring during the operation is of great importance. This usually includes oximetry, respiratory rate, electrocardiogram, non-invasive and intra-arterial blood pressure, end-tidal carbon dioxide, bispectral index, and urinary output.

Patients are usually placed in supine or semi-lateral position. This enables them to see the anesthesiologist's face clearly, enhance face-to-face communication, and alleviate anxiety during the awake phase. It also facilitates access to the patient's face and neck, which is important for airway management should any crisis develop. Drapes used for the sterile field should be clear and fixed with clips and bands to the sides to avoid blinding the patient's view and to promote face-to-face interaction, thus minimizing the risk of claustrophobia. Contrary to other surgical procedures, eye ointment should not be administered, as it can blur the patient's vision during the awake phase.

During the entire surgery, the head is properly fixed in a head frame. This is important from the anesthesiologist's view for two reasons. First, the pain in the pin hole area in the awake phase is increased, especially when the duration of surgery is extended, and the effect of local anesthetic agents diminishes. Therefore, if the Mayfield is used, application of adequate local anesthesia should be considered before pin insertion. Second, it restricts the head and neck movement, which is vital in airway management. Of note, the duration of the awake phase should be reduced as much as possible because of the risk of diminished anesthetic agent effects and discomfort of remaining in a fixed position.

The operating room should not be crowded, and unnecessary noise should be kept at a minimum. This can contribute immensely to reducing patient anxiety. Similar to other awake operations, patient comfort and relaxation during the awake phase along with the functional language test is of extreme importance, and any disturbance of their tranquility can lead to failure of the procedure. Adequate operating table padding, and comfortable head, neck, and leg positioning leads to better cooperation between the patient and the team. In fact, in some neurosurgical centers, the patient's position (i.e., supine, lateral, or semi-lateral) is inspected and adjusted the day before surgery. However, when the lesion is in the occipital area or visual cortex, a sitting position is usually preferred. A typical layout for the theater is shown in Fig. 1. Room temperature should also be adjusted for maximizing patient comfort and cooperation during the awake phase [2].

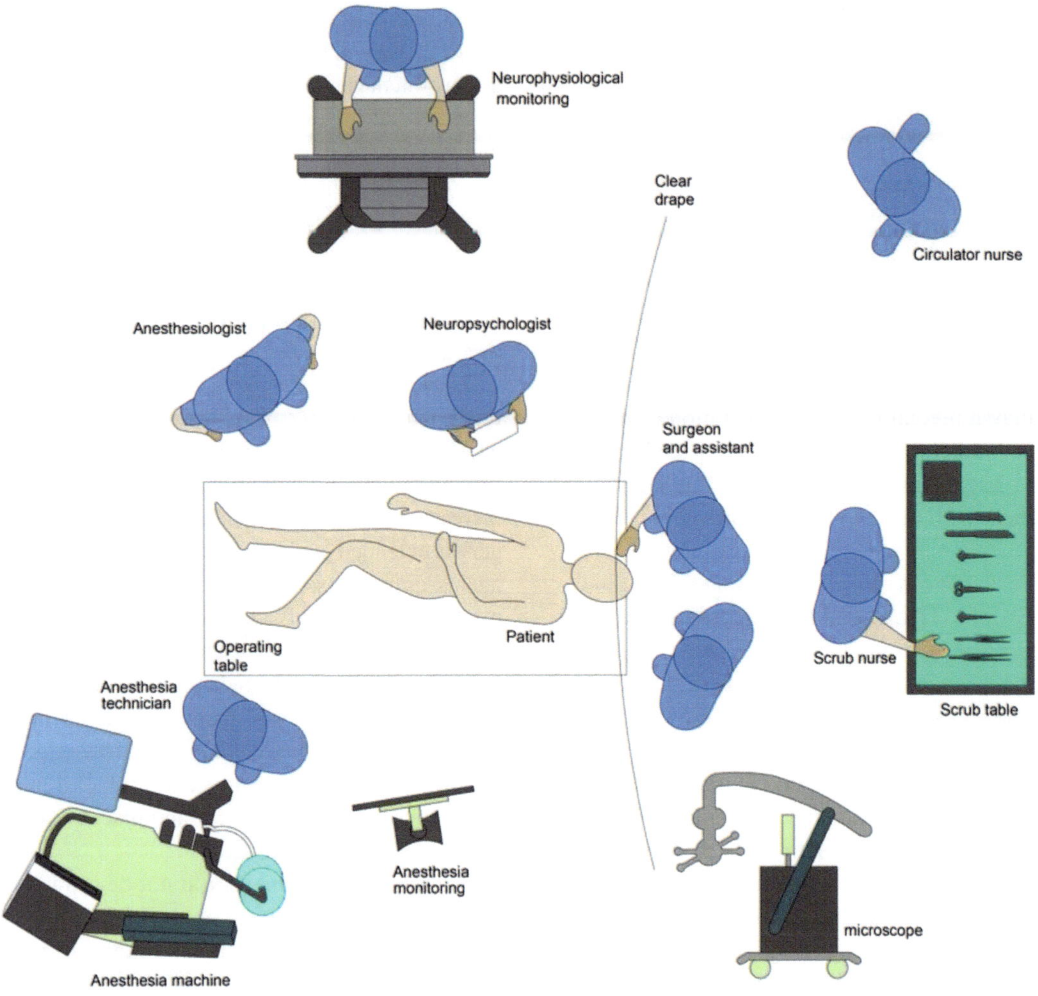

Fig. 1 Surgical team schema

7 Anesthesia Management, Approaches, and Principles

The most challenging aspect of anesthesia in awake craniotomy is choosing the right anesthetic technique. Although certain techniques are conventionally employed in most centers, there is no consensus about a predefined set of guidelines which should be followed. This emphasizes the need for further research on anesthesia technique, and how the procedure should be modified to adapt to any particular patient and situation.

Premedicating patients prior to anesthesia induction is an option; however, the use of this for awake craniotomy is not common, and it is only considered for patients with acid reflux problems and those who take steroids, anti-hypertensive, or anti-epileptic medications. These medications should be taken as prescribed on the day of surgery. If the patient is on anti-convulsant medications, plasma levels should be measured the day before the operation [2]. Generally, the drugs administered prior to surgery include antiemetics and prophylactic antibiotics which are prescribed for prevention of infection at the surgical site. Common antiemetics used in awake craniotomy are ondansetron and dexamethasone, and the latter can also decrease brain edema during surgery.

Paracetamol and non-steroidal anti-inflammatory drugs (NSAIDs) may also be used to control pain. Painful procedures (such as insertion of the urinary catheter, large-bore IV access, and arterial line insertion) should be carried out when the patient is sedated or asleep. Since urinary catheterization causes discomfort in the awake phase, usually a smaller size is inserted under sedation (or not used at all). Sterile intra-urethral viscous lidocaine gel application can also alleviate patient discomfort [24]. It is emphasized that restricted fluid replacement should be given to patients who can not tolerate a urinary catheter.

In addition to standard monitoring, other means of monitoring may be used. Bispectral index monitoring (BIS) method, which monitors the depth of anesthesia, is used in awake craniotomy. Several studies have reported that the use of BIS can decrease the required dose of anesthetic medications and shorten the time needed to awake patients for the mapping phase [25]. Capnography is also used to monitor patient ventilation and carbon-dioxide level. Considering its wide application as a basic monitoring in anesthesia, this technique is commonly used (especially during the mapping phase) to ensure adequate ventilation when the patient is not completely awake [2].

Although anesthesia regimens and drug doses vary in different techniques, a general set of principles are followed in all of them, such as aiming at enhancing patients' hemodynamic stability, promoting comfort, preventing nausea, vomiting, pain, establishing control of level of consciousness, and providing adequate ventilation. There are generally three main anesthetic approaches: sedation, asleep-awake-asleep, and asleep-awake. It should be noted, however, that there is no consensus about the right anesthetic technique, and different methods are used according to the surgeon's preference, pathology of the lesion, duration of the surgery, and the patient's cooperation.

Regardless of the anesthesia technique, scalp block is crucial in the awake craniotomy. In some cases, scalp block (also known as regional block or scalp anesthetization) which includes the injection of a local anesthetic to the locations of seven nerves on either sides), is the only analgesia method [2]. Providing an adequate dose of local anesthetics for nerve block, and additionally the area of pins, the field, and dura block is of critical importance. Cutaneous nerves (which stem from different branches of trigeminal and cervical spinal nerves) innervate the skin, periosteum, and pericranium of the outer table of the skull [2]. Efficient analgesia through scalp block stabilizes hemodynamics, which can be disturbed due to the painful stimuli stress response. Scalp block is considered as an anatomical block which is quite different from a ring block. In the ring block, large amounts of local anesthetics are used which can cause toxicity without deeply anesthetizing fascia temporalis. Nonetheless, the brain tissue itself is not sensitive to pain and needs no anesthesia.

Since patients are awake and all IV analgesics are stopped, their tolerance of pain depends on the efficacy of the regional and field blocks. Scalp block is essential during neurocognitive testing and functional mapping when sedation and analgesia are at their minimum levels. In addition, as local anesthetics are used prior to pinning the patient's head in the Mayfield, sometimes the scalp block may not be done, but most anesthesiologists prefer to perform a bilateral scalp block before pinning [2].

The dose of local anesthetics should be calculated for each individual patient. When extra doses of local anesthetics are used during infiltrating temporalis fascia, the skin, and dura mater, the choice and dose of the local anesthetics should be monitored and recorded. Different concentrations of lidocaine, bupivacaine, levobupivacaine, and ropivacaine are generally used as local anesthetics for scalp block [20]. Epinephrine 1:200,000 is usually added to local anesthetics and provides different benefits, including: increasing the dose of anesthetics that can safely be used, decreasing local bleeding, and maximizing the duration of analgesia. However, since systemic absorption of epinephrine may lead to tachycardia and hypertension, it should be used in moderation.

7.1 Scalp Block

Regardless of the type of anesthesia, regional block is essential to control pain. Scalp block usually is performed after induction of anesthesia, but in certain circumstances, it may be carried out with the sedation process (e.g., functional neurosurgery with mild sedation). Depending on the side of surgery and whether or not Mayfield is used, regional block can be conducted unilaterally or bilaterally (performed bilaterally when Mayfield is used). The location of scalp block is usually at seven different sites, which are at the branches of the cutaneous nerve supplying the innervation of the scalp. At each site, 2–5 cc of local anesthetic is injected, and aspiration is mandatory to ensure that the anesthetic is not delivered inadvertently into a vein or artery. These nerves are elaborated as follows:

Supraorbital nerve is a branch of the V1 (ophthalmic) and the first truncation of the trigeminal nerve. It innervates the forehead, the upper eyelid, anterior part of the scalp, and top part of the head, and then extends to the lambdoidal suture. The best method for finding and blocking this nerve is palpating the supraorbital notch, inserting the needle at this location vertically, and injecting the local anesthetic [2].

Supratrochlear nerve is a branch of the V1 division of the trigeminal nerve which supplies sensory innervation to the forehead and skin of the lower part of it near the midline, conjunctiva, and upper eyelid. To block this nerve, a local anesthetic should be injected medial to the supraorbital notch between the notch and the bridge of the nose [26].

Zygomaticotemporal nerve is a branch of the V2 division of the trigeminal nerve. It is a small nerve in the face which innervates a small area of the forehead and temporal area. In this location, anesthetics are injected from the supraorbital ridge to the posterior segment of the zygomatic arch. It should be noted, however, that injection should be deep and superficial to the temporalis muscle [27].

Auriculotemporal nerve is a branch of the V3 division of the trigeminal nerve which innervates the auricle, temporal areas, lower face, lower lip, and the supra-auricular scalp. The auriculotemporal nerve is usually blocked by injection over the zygomatic process 1–1.5 cm anterior to the ear at the same level as the tragus. It is important to mention that the superficial temporal artery is anterior to the auriculotemporal nerve in this location, and it should be palpated before the blockade [27]. Moreover, the injection should not be carried out below the zygoma because of the risk of transient facial paralysis.

Greater occipital nerve is a branch of the second cervical spinal nerve, and it innervates the posterior part of the scalp to the top of the head and over the auricle [2]. For effectively blocking this nerve, the needle should be inserted medial to the occipital artery which is located between occipital protuberance and mastoid process [28].

Lesser occipital nerve (small occipital nerve) is a cutaneous spinal nerve and a branch of C2 or C3 from the cervical plexus. It ascends along the posterior border of the sternocleidomastoid muscle and innervates the skin of the posterior of the auricle, mastoid region, and scalp of the lateral side of the head. This nerve can be blocked by inserting the needle just after the lateral third of a line between the external occipital protuberance and lower end of the mastoid process [29].

Greater auricular nerve is the largest superficial branch of the cervical plexus which lies deep underneath the platysma muscle and ascends the neck over the surface of the sternocleidomastoid muscle. This nerve has two branches and provides sensation to the ear, mastoid process, parotid, and the mandible angle. To block this nerve, first the level of tragus is marked and the local anesthetic should be infiltrated about 2 cm posterior to the auricle [2].

For an effective scalp block, the patient's position should be comfortable, and the procedure should be carried out at least 20 min prior to the skin incision so that the anesthesiologist can be confident that the required level of analgesia has been achieved and can monitor the patient for any potential toxicity or complication attributable to the anesthetic. This procedure is usually carried out using bupivacaine 0.25–0.5% mixed with epinephrine 1:200,000 using sterile gloves and a 25-gauge needle to ensure safe and adequate

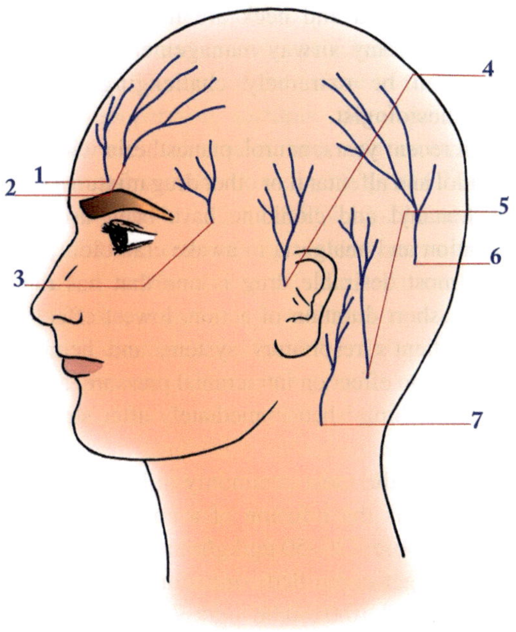

Fig. 2 Scalp block; (1) Supratrochlear nerve, (2) Supraorbital nerve, (3) Zygomaticotemporal nerve, (4) Auriculotemporal nerve, (5) Lesser occipital nerve, (6) Greater occipital nerve, (7) Greater auricular nerve

analgesia for approximately 6–8 h (bupivacaine 0.375% is usually favored for scalp block). In addition, because the dura is highly innervated, it should be anesthetized through infiltration of a local anesthetic around the nerve trunk (which runs along the middle meningeal artery). A field block is carried out around the edges of the craniotomy by lidocaine 1% as a fast-acting agent. The dura also can be anesthetized through infiltration of lidocaine with epinephrine between its leaves [24]. To avoid toxicity, the anesthesiologist should calculate and determine the total dose and volume of local anesthetics (Fig. 2).

7.2 General Anesthesia Induction

In the 'asleep/awake ± asleep' technique, the patient is awake during neurocognitive testing and intraoperative mapping. The first asleep phase is started with general anesthesia induction, which is supported by airway protection with a supraglottic device or endotracheal tube.

Although stimulation of the brain tissue itself is not painful, several procedures can disturb the patient's comfort level and inflict pain, such as the scalp block, fixing the Mayfield, craniotomy, scalp, and dura mater incision. Therefore, the procedure should initially begin with induction of general anesthesia. There is no consensus about the drug of choice at this stage, but generally, it is advisable that the dose of drugs should be smaller in comparison with other operations to minimize the time for awakening the patient and encouraging cooperation. In centers where awake craniotomy procedures are regularly carried out, the time needed for scalp removal, preparation of the brain field for intraoperative mapping, and tumor resection are usually estimated by the anesthesiology team. The duration of the operation should be clarified by the surgeon so that the anesthesiologist can select the medication and dose accordingly.

Prior to the emergence of the awake phase, anesthesia medications should be decreased or discontinued. For example, 10–15 min before awakening the patient, the propofol infusion is stopped, and the dose of remifentanil is reduced. The airway device should be removed only after monitoring the upper airway reflexes or passing the emergence stage of anesthesia if it is deemed to be safe. After the awake phase is completed or the tumor is completely resected, general anesthesia should be induced, and the airway device should be replaced. Nonetheless, in certain circumstances, the awake phase is maintained until the end of the operation. One advantage of this approach is preventing hypoventilation and carbon dioxide accumulation, which may increase intracranial pressure. In addition, the depth of anesthesia in the noxious parts of the procedure can be controlled more effectively.

Propofol and remifentanil infusion are commonly used in awake craniotomy [30]. Anesthetic volatiles such as sevoflurane may also be used, but they can interfere with neurological monitoring. If dexmedetomidine is used in this method, it is preferred in the awake and scalp closure phases. Inserting an airway device for the patient intraoperatively could become challenging in a semi-lateral position when the patient's head and ment team summoned; all infusions discontinued; the patient's ventilation maintained with a bag mask at 100% oxygen using the jaw thrust maneuver, and an oral or nasal airway should be inserted. In life-threatening situations, laryngeal mask airway (LMA), an endotracheal tube, and a video laryngoscope should be considered. In case of mask ventilation failure, insertion of an LMA is generally required. Pulling the tongue out using a gauze swab or a Magill forceps can be a helpful maneuver in this situation which can facilitate LMA insertion. Despite all efforts for LMA insertion, intubation using a flexible fiberoptic device or a video laryngoscope can be an alternative [24].

Moreover, if the patient vomits during the operation for any reason (such as anesthesia agents or stimulation of the gag reflex which may occur after extubation or removing the LMA), it can be extremely difficult to immediately adjust the patient's head to a lateral position. If vomiting occurs, the risk of aspiration from gastric contents can create a critical situation for both patient and anesthesiologist.

Hypoventilation, hypercapnia, airway obstruction, apnea, and hypoxia may happen during the awake phase of the operation; therefore, the patient's respiratory condition should be closely monitored. Another uncommon situation is the need for conversion to general anesthesia. This usually occurs when respiratory complications cannot be controlled through the aforementioned means and respiratory distress develops despite all the airway opening interventions. The risk of pulmonary aspiration exists, especially when patients complain of nausea. Although awake craniotomy is performed under low-level sedation, hemodynamic parameters are more manageable in this technique in comparison with general anesthesia, but cardiovascular complications such as hypertension, hypotension, bradycardia, and tachycardia are sometimes reported.

Managing the level of sedation is of key importance during the awake phase and either inadequate or excessive sedation can lead to failure of the procedure. Inadequate sedation can trigger pain and discomfort mainly due to the positioning of the patient. In contrast, a high dose of sedatives may lead to nausea, vomiting, or both, and interfere with patient cooperation. Scalp blocks should be carried out at least 20 min before starting the incision to avoid local anesthetic toxicity [20]. As previously mentioned, detection and addressing psychological issues prior to the operation is vital. Patient's anxiety, agitation, intolerance of the procedure, and fatigue can all interfere with the necessary assessments during the awake phase.

Seizure activity is another common complication (3–16%) which sometimes occurs during the brain mapping phase. It can usually be treated with irrigation of the brain tissue using ice-saline several times as necessary, and most seizures can be controlled by iced cortical spray. However, in patients who do not respond to this treatment, IV propofol (30–50 mg) should be administered repeatedly as needed. Other agents, such as benzodiazepines, anticonvulsants, or deep sedatives, may also be used [24]. Patients with a history of seizures are generally more at risk during the brain tissue stimulation phase. Therefore, if there is any history of seizure or anticonvulsant use, management should be initiated or planned prior to the start of the procedure. For some reasons such as, prolonged immobilization and having an unpleasant sensation of a Foley catheter in urethra, the awake phase maybe intolerable for the patient. A detailed list of intraoperative adverse events is tabulated in Table 3.

Table 3 Intraoperative complications

Respiratory	Hypoventilation
	Apnea
	Hypercapnia
	Airway obstruction
	Hypoxia
	Conversion to GA
	Aspiration
Cardiovascular	Hypertension
	Hypotension
	Tachycardia
	Bradycardia
Anesthetic techniques and drugs	Level of sedation (too deep, too light…)
	Inadequate pain control
	Nausea and vomiting
	Local anesthetic toxicity
Neurological	Seizure
Psychological factors	Anxiety
	Agitation
	Tiredness

10 Closure

After completion of brain mapping and tumor resection phase, the anesthesiologist should choose the most suitable method for anesthesia during the closure stage according to the situation and patient's condition. As closure of the dura matter, the bone flap and the scalp can be painful, the patient should be well-sedated and calm but re-anesthetizing or re-inserting of the airway device is not usually necessary. Because of the fatigue caused by the awake phase and less painful stimuli in the closure in comparison with the opening phase, patients usually need a lower dose of infused sedatives [24]. Moreover, the patient should be awakened gently and calmly without any incidence of coughing to avoid increased intracranial pressure.

11 Postoperative Care

Postoperatively, the patients' condition should be monitored in neurosurgery ward or in the intensive care unit. In some centers, all patients are admitted in neuro- intensive care unit for overnight monitoring. Hematoma can develop during the first six hours after surgery. Routine postoperative imaging can be of great assistance as it can identify any expansion of a possible hematoma and other adverse complications within 48 hours after the procedure [2]. Systemic pain relivers (such as paracetamol, opioids, NSAIDS) can be used after surgery to control pain. It is usually recommended to do scalp block preoperatively to facilitate postoperative pain control, although pain relivers are usually necessary as the duration of block is short.

12 Conclusion

The advantage of precise complete tumor removal in awake craniotomy can reduce potential complications and increase overall patient survival and satisfaction [32, 33]. In a study of over 1000 patients who underwent the procedure, a low rate of mortality and morbidity was reported. Therefore, awake craniotomy can be considered as a safe well-tolerated procedure with low risk of failure or need for conversion to general anesthesia. As new neurosurgery techniques and technologies emerge, anesthesiologists should continue to broaden their knowledge in this area. Obviously, anesthesia for awake patients using this technique is critical and requires more caution and care in comparison to conventional surgical procedures. Although no standard technique of anesthesia has been established yet, more RCTs are needed to establish a guideline for a particular method in anesthesia induction for awake craniotomy. Moreover, there is a need for long-term studies concerning tumor recurrence, survival, and the quality of life of patients. Determining the best method for maximizing patient cooperation and comfort through the selection of appropriate anesthetic drugs, and their dosages to induce the required level of anesthesia during the awake phase are equally important.

References

1. Hassan WMNW. The history of awake craniotomy in Hospital Universiti Sains Malaysia. Malays J Med Sci. 2013;20(5):67.
2. Burnand C, Sebastian J. Anaesthesia for awake craniotomy. Continuing Educ Anaesth Crit Care Pain. 2013;14(1):6–11.
3. Kim SH, Choi SH. Anesthetic considerations for awake craniotomy. Anesth Pain Med. 2020;15(3):269.
4. Gerritsen JKW, Arends L, Klimek M, Dirven CMF, Vincent AJ-PE. Impact of intraoperative stimulation mapping on high-grade glioma surgery outcome: a meta-analysis. Acta Neurochir. 2019;161(1):99–107.
5. Eseonu CI, Rincon-Torroella J, ReFaey K, Lee YM, Nangiana J, Vivas-Buitrago T, et al. Awake craniotomy vs craniotomy under general anesthesia for perirolandic gliomas: evaluating perioperative complications and extent of resection. Neurosurgery. 2017;81(3):481–9.
6. Zhang K, Gelb AW. Awake craniotomy: indications, benefits, and techniques. Colomb J Anestesiol. 2018;46:46–51.
7. Adams F. The extant works of aretaeus: the cappadocian. London: Sydenham Society; 1856.
8. Frost EA. A history of neuroanesthesia. In: The wondrous story of anesthesia. New York: Springer; 2014. p. 871–85.
9. Froeschner EH. Two examples of ancient skull surgery. J Neurosurg. 1992;76(3):550–2.
10. Monira KM, Munan SM. Review on Datura metel: a potential medicinal plant. Glob J Res Med Plants Indig Med. 2012;1(4):123.

operative tasks as well as intraoperative stress and anxiety, although there have been reports on successful implementation of AC in this patient population [20–24]. Patient willingness to undergo AC is of utmost importance for success. Moreover, obstructive sleep apnea, low tolerance to pain, obesity, and chronic cough or wheezing constitute the other contraindications [6]. (For a full discussion on pre-operative considerations in AC, please see "Patient Selection for Awake Craniotomy<Patient Selection, Awake Craniotomy>").

3 Intraoperative Task Selection

The intraoperative tasks should correspond to the cortical and subcortical areas that will be encountered during surgery [11, 25]. These are determined prior to surgery and must be agreed upon by the surgeon and the tester (e.g., speech therapist, neuropsychologist, resident, or anesthesiologist) [4, 14, 26]. These are typically rehearsed with the patient at least 1 day prior to AC [27]. As most AC is done for language and motor mapping, we usually test at least object naming and semantic association with concomitant contralateral arm movement, elbow flexion, and opening and closing of the fist during the initial phases. These serve to assess language and motor functions, as well as enabling the patient to "warm up" to the process of AC. Dealing with "non-language" areas uses different tests accustomed to patient function [8, 13, 28, 29]. In general, bimanual coordination tasks for the supplementary motor area [30, 31], visual field assessment for visual pathway mapping [32–34], spatial cognition for temporo-parietal mapping [35, 36], somatosensory and calculation for parietal mapping [37, 38], judgment for pre-frontal mapping [39, 40], emotion and mentalizing for insular mapping [41, 42]; are used to name a few. (Fig. 1) Subcortical structures must also be considered during task preparation such as assessing semantic association and face-based mentalizing for the inferior fronto-occipital fasciculus [43, 44]. We follow a 4-second interval in between items for each task, as faster lexical access speed has been found to improve functional outcomes in AC with brain mapping [45].

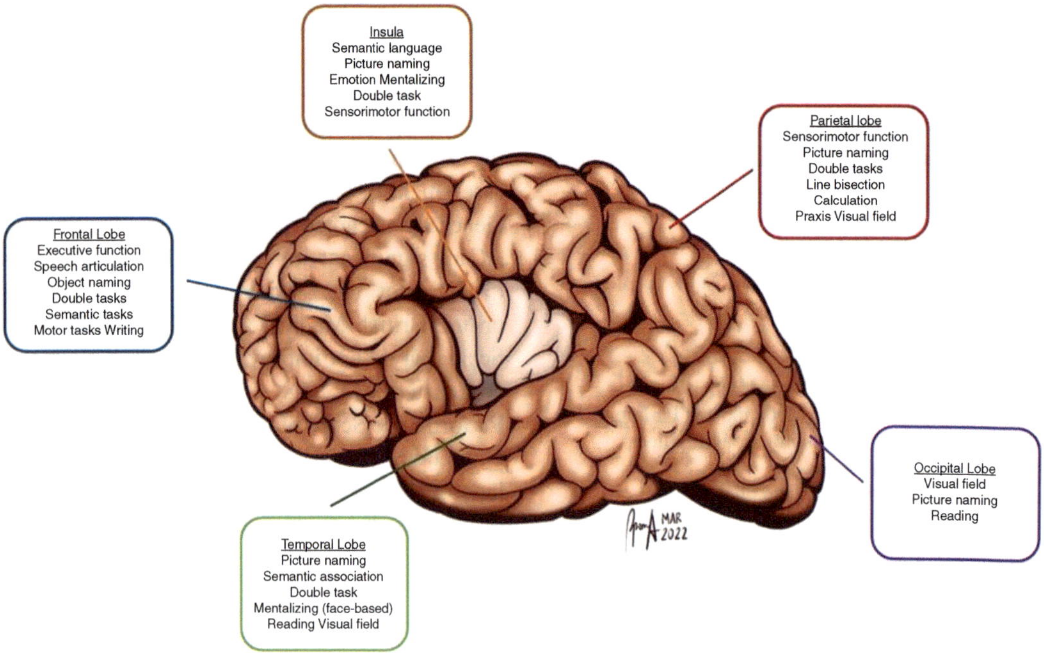

Fig. 1 Schematic diagram of cortical anatomy with possible intraoperative tasks (figure courtesy of Dr. Almira Apor)

4 Conduct of Surgery and Intraoperative Mapping

Despite many centers that apply the asleep-awake-asleep technique for awake surgery, in our institution, we employ the asleep-awake technique [46]. The AC set-up for the operating room differs from the usual in that ample space is allotted near the patient's face and arms to facilitate intraoperative testing [47]. The patient is positioned either supine with the head turned, without straining the neck (jugular veins not distended); or in a full lateral position with an axillary pad for comfort; pending the location of the craniotomy [48, 49]. After induction of anesthesia, or under laryngeal mask airway, the skin is cleansed and scrubbed with 7.5% iodine solution then prepped with 10% iodine solution [46]. The AC drape consists of either sterile transparent plastic sheet, providing the surgeon more visibility during intraoperative testing; or opaque drapes that are used particularly in institutions with a video camera or microphone [50]. An additional stand is positioned in line with the patient's head in order to secure the drape and create a tent wherein the tester and patient are performing the intraoperative task. This prevents the drape from obstructing the patient's view [14, 46]. Some institutions prefer to hang the sterile drape over two tall intravenous (IV) stands beside the OR bed, thus naturally creating space for intraoperative testing on the anesthesia side [51]. The main idea for draping is to establish an area for the patient and examiner to do intraoperative tasks comfortably.

Skin and soft tissue opening, and craniotomy are performed classically with the patient not fully awake. Prior to entering the dura, it is infiltrated with lidocaine 2%, targeted along the branches of the middle meningeal artery if it is visible, and along the dural opening [52]. Anesthetic infiltration of the dura must be emphasized as it is highly sensitive to pain since it is innervated by the trigeminal nerve [53]. The patient is then awakened prior to dural opening to prevent brain herniation in the event that the patient coughs [11, 54]. It should be noted that the testing team (i.e., speech therapist, neuropsychologist, neurosurgery resident, or neuro-anesthesiologist) must already be present in the room once the dura is exposed.

Upon awakening, the patient is reoriented to the operating room to avoid feelings of apprehension [55]. Anxiety may arise from the unfamiliarity of the operating room setup as well as the limited visualization due to the drapes, among other things [56]. It is of utmost importance to provide reassurance and comfort as a relaxed patient can facilitate intraoperative testing [57]. Discomfort may be felt from an uncomfortable position, restricted movements from the head clamp or straps, as well as unnoticed pressure points [58, 59]. These issues should be resolved by the operating room team through calm explanation and consoling [55].

Baseline orientation, language, and motor functions are tested upon awakening. These tasks usually consist of requesting the patient to count from 1 to 10, basic orientating questions (name, age), and movement of target extremities such as the contralateral arm and leg [60]. Once baseline functioning has been assessed, cortical stimulation and brain mapping may commence. Majority of cortical mapping is for language and motor tasks [61, 62]. As such, we employ concomitant tasks [63] with constant elbow flexion-extension and opening-closing of the contralateral arm as the patient identifies objects using a widely used neuropsychological assessment tool (Boston Naming Test in our setting) [46, 64]. Cortical stimulator settings used are classical: frequency 60 Hertz, duration 1 millisecond, current starting at 0.5 mA increasing by 0.5 mA up to 6 mA [11, 65]. For institutions without electrocorticography to detect after-discharges, we recommend not increasing the frequency above 3 mA to reduce the frequency of intraoperative seizures, in accordance with Boetto and colleagues [66]. Positive sites are deemed as such when the errors occur 2 or 3 times [8]. These cortical sites are labeled and noted by the surgeon and the circulating nurse. The labels can be small numbered and lettered pieces of paper or any type of labeling material. In our institution, due to the unavailability of the commercial labels, we tend to use cut pieces of the cardboard from the sterile gown (Fig. 2).

11. Hervey-jumper SL, Li J, Lau D, et al. Awake craniotomy to maximize glioma resection: methods and technical nuances over a 27-year period. J Neurosurg. 2015;123(2):325–39. https://doi.org/10.3171/2014.10.JNS141520.Disclosure.
12. De Witt Hamer PC, Klein M, Hervey-Jumper SL, Wefel JS, Berger MS. Functional outcomes and health-related quality of life following glioma surgery. Neurosurgery. 2021;88(4):720–32. https://doi.org/10.1093/neuros/nyaa365.
13. Kim SS, McCutcheon IE, Suki D, et al. Awake craniotomy for brain tumors near eloquent cortex: correlation of intraoperative cortical mapping with neurological outcomes in 309 consecutive patients. Neurosurgery. 2009;64(5):836–45. https://doi.org/10.1227/01.NEU.0000342405.80881.81.
14. Benyaich Z, Hajhouji F, Laghmari M, et al. Awake craniotomy with functional mapping for glioma resection in a limited-resource-setting: preliminary experience from a lower-middle income country. World Neurosurg. 2020;139:200–7. https://doi.org/10.1016/j.wneu.2020.04.039.
15. Southwell DG, Hervey-jumper SL, Perry DW, Berger MS. Intraoperative mapping during repeat awake craniotomy reveals the functional plasticity of adult cortex. J Neurosurg. 2016;124(5):1460–9. https://doi.org/10.3171/2015.5.JNS142833.
16. Sanai N, Mirzadeh Z, Berger MS. Functional outcome after language mapping for glioma resection. N Engl J Med. 2008;358(1):18–27. https://doi.org/10.1056/nejmoa067819.
17. Sanai N, Berger MS. Glioma extent of resection and its impact on patient outcome. Neurosurgery. 2009;65(4):229–35. https://doi.org/10.1227/01.NEU.0000310769.20996.BD.
18. Dziedzic T, Bernstein M. Awake craniotomy for brain tumor: indications, technique and benefits. Expert Rev Neurother. 2014;14(12):1405–15. https://doi.org/10.1586/14737175.2014.979793.
19. Hill CS, Severgnini F, McKintosh E. How I do it: awake craniotomy. Acta Neurochir. 2017;159(1):173–6. https://doi.org/10.1007/s00701-016-3021-z.
20. Delion M, Terminassian A, Lehousse T, et al. Specificities of awake craniotomy and brain mapping in children for resection of supratentorial tumors in the language area. World Neurosurg. 2015;84(6):1645–52. https://doi.org/10.1016/j.wneu.2015.06.073.
21. Lohkamp LN, Mottolese C, Szathmari A, et al. Awake brain surgery in children—review of the literature and state-of-the-art. Childs Nerv Syst. 2019;35(11):2071–7. https://doi.org/10.1007/s00381-019-04279-w.
22. Balogun JA, Khan OH, Taylor M, et al. Pediatric awake craniotomy and intra-operative stimulation mapping. J Clin Neurosci. 2014;21(11):1891–4. https://doi.org/10.1016/j.jocn.2014.07.013.
23. Alcaraz García-Tejedor G, Echániz G, Strantzas S, et al. Feasibility of awake craniotomy in the pediatric population. Paediatr Anaesth. 2020;30(4):480–9. https://doi.org/10.1111/pan.13833.
24. Akay A, Rüken M, Çetin HY, Seval HÖ, Lekel S. Pediatric awake craniotomy for brain lesions. Pediatr Neurosurg. 2016;51(2):103–8. https://doi.org/10.1159/000442988.
25. Coello AF, Moritz-Gasser S, Martino J, Martinoni M, Matsuda R, Duffau H. Selection of intraoperative tasks for awake mapping based on relationships between tumor location and functional networks: a review. J Neurosurg. 2013;119(6):1380–94. https://doi.org/10.3171/2013.6.JNS122470.
26. Leal RTM, Barcellos BM, Landeiro JA. Technical aspects of awake craniotomy with mapping for brain tumors in a limited resource setting. World Neurosurg. 2018;113:67–72. https://doi.org/10.1016/j.wneu.2018.02.013.
27. De Benedictis A, Moritz-Gasser S, Duffau H. Awake mapping optimizes the extent of resection for low-grade gliomas in eloquent areas. Neurosurgery. 2010;66(6):1074–84. https://doi.org/10.1227/01.NEU.0000369514.74284.78.
28. Sellier A, Moritz-Gasser S, Lemaitre AL, Herbet G, Duffau H. Presence of a translator in the operating theater for awake mapping in foreign patients with low-grade glioma: a surgical experience based on 18 different native languages. J Neurosurg. 2021;135(2):496–504. https://doi.org/10.3171/2020.6.JNS201071.
29. Morshed R, Young J, Lee A, Hervey-Jumper S. Functional mapping for glioma surgery, part 2: intraoperative mapping tools. Neurosurg Clin N Am. 2021;32(1):75–81. https://doi.org/10.1016/j.nec.2020.09.001.
30. Klitsinikos D, Ekert JO, Carels A, Samandouras G. Mapping and anatomo-surgical techniques for SMA-cingulum-corpus callosum gliomas; how I do it. Acta Neurochir. 2021;163(5):1239–46. https://doi.org/10.1007/s00701-021-04774-7.
31. Shibata S, Yamao Y, Kunieda T, et al. Intraoperative electrophysiologic mapping of medial frontal motor areas and functional outcomes. World Neurosurg. 2020;138:e389–404. https://doi.org/10.1016/j.wneu.2020.02.129.
32. Sarubbo S, De Benedictis A, Milani P, et al. The course and the anatomo-functional relationships of the optic radiation: a combined study with "post mortem" dissections and "in vivo" direct electrical mapping. J Anat. 2015;226(1):47–59. https://doi.org/10.1111/joa.12254.
33. Nguyen HS, Sundaram SV, Mosier KM, Cohen-Gadol AA. A method to map the visual cortex during an awake craniotomy: technical note. J Neurosurg. 2011;114(4):922–6. https://doi.org/10.3171/2010.11.JNS101293.
34. Shahar T, Korn A, Barkay G, et al. Elaborate mapping of the posterior visual pathway in awake craniotomy. J Neurosurg. 2018;128(5):1503–11. https://doi.org/10.3171/2017.2.JNS162757.
35. Roux FE, Dufor O, Lauwers-Cances V, et al. Electrostimulation mapping of spatial neglect.

Neurosurgery. 2011;69(6):1218–31. https://doi.org/10.1227/NEU.0b013e31822aefd2.

36. Nakada M, Nakajima R, Okita H, et al. Awake surgery for right frontal lobe glioma can preserve visuospatial cognition and spatial working memory. J Neuro-Oncol. 2021;151(2):221–30. https://doi.org/10.1007/s11060-020-03656-9.
37. Breshears JD, Gaona CM, Roland JL, et al. Mapping sensorimotor cortex with slow cortical potential resting-state networks while awake and under anesthesia. Neurosurgery. 2012;71(2):305–16. https://doi.org/10.1227/NEU.0b013e318258e5d1.
38. Della PA, De Pellegrin S, Lazzarini A, et al. Subcortical mapping of calculation processing in the right parietal lobe. J Neurosurg. 2015;122(5):1038–41. https://doi.org/10.3171/2014.10.JNS14261.
39. Plaza M, Gatignol P, Cohen H, Berger B, Duffau H. A discrete area within the left dorsolateral prefrontal cortex involved in visual-verbal incongruence judgment. Cereb Cortex. 2008;18(6):1253–9. https://doi.org/10.1093/cercor/bhm169.
40. Duffau H. The " frontal syndrome" revisited: lessons from electrostimulation mapping studies. Cortex. 2012;48(1):120–31. https://doi.org/10.1016/j.cortex.2011.04.029.
41. Yordanova YN, Cochereau J, Duffau H, Herbet G. Combining resting state functional MRI with intraoperative cortical stimulation to map the mentalizing network. NeuroImage. 2019;186:628–36. https://doi.org/10.1016/j.neuroimage.2018.11.046.
42. Nakajima R, Yordanova YN, Duffau H, Herbet G. Neuropsychological evidence for the crucial role of the right arcuate fasciculus in the face-based mentalizing network: a disconnection analysis. Neuropsychologia. 2018;115(January):179–87. https://doi.org/10.1016/j.neuropsychologia.2018.01.024.
43. Yordanova YN, Duffau H, Herbet G. Neural pathways subserving face-based mentalizing. Brain Struct Funct. 2017;222(7):3087–105. https://doi.org/10.1007/s00429-017-1388-0.
44. Chenin L, Lefranc M, Velut S, Foulon P, Havet E, Peltier J. Cortical and subcortical functional neuroanatomy for low-grade glioma surgery. Neurochirurgie. 2017;63(3):117–21. https://doi.org/10.1016/j.neuchi.2016.10.001.
45. Moritz-Gasser S, Herbet G, Maldonado IL, Duffau H. Lexical access speed is significantly correlated with the return to professional activities after awake surgery for low-grade gliomas. J Neuro-Oncol. 2012;107(3):633–41. https://doi.org/10.1007/s11060-011-0789-9.
46. Pascual JSG, Omar AT, Gaddi MJS, et al. Awake craniotomy in low-resource settings: findings from a retrospective cohort in The Philippines. World Neurosurg. 2021;145:500–507.e1. https://doi.org/10.1016/j.wneu.2020.10.070.
47. Gogos AJ, Young JS, Morshed RA, Hervey-Jumper SL, Berger MS. Awake glioma surgery: technical evolution and nuances. J Neuro-Oncol. 2020;147(3):515–24. https://doi.org/10.1007/s11060-020-03482-z.
48. Lima GLO, Dezamis E, Corns R, et al. Surgical resection of incidental diffuse gliomas involving eloquent brain areas. Rationale, functional, epileptological and oncological outcomes. Neurochirurgie. 2017;63(3):250–8. https://doi.org/10.1016/j.neuchi.2016.08.007.
49. Beez T, Boge K, Wager M, et al. Tolerance of awake surgery for glioma: a prospective European low grade glioma network multicenter study. Acta Neurochir. 2013;155(7):1301–8. https://doi.org/10.1007/s00701-013-1759-0.
50. Szelényi A, Bello L, Duffau H, et al. Intraoperative electrical stimulation in awake craniotomy: methodological aspects of current practice. Neurosurg Focus. 2010;28(2):1–8. https://doi.org/10.3171/2009.12.FOCUS09237.
51. Ng S, Herbet G, Moritz-Gasser S, Duffau H. Return to work following surgery for incidental diffuse low-grade glioma: a prospective series with 74 patients. Neurosurgery. 2020;87(4):720–9. https://doi.org/10.1093/neuros/nyz513.
52. Fontaine D, Almairac F, Santucci S, et al. Dural and pial pain-sensitive structures in humans: new inputs from awake craniotomies. Brain. 2018;141(4):1040–8. https://doi.org/10.1093/brain/awy005.
53. Fontaine D, Almairac F. Pain during awake craniotomy for brain tumor resection. Incidence, causes, consequences and management. Neurochirurgie. 2017;63(3):204–7. https://doi.org/10.1016/j.neuchi.2016.08.005.
54. Arzoine J, Levé C, Pérez-Hick A, et al. Anesthesia management for low-grade glioma awake surgery: a European low-grade glioma network survey. Acta Neurochir. 2020;162(7):1701–7. https://doi.org/10.1007/s00701-020-04274-0.
55. Colgan DD, Eddy A, Aulet-Leon M, et al. Compassion, communication, and the perception of control: a mixed methods study to investigate patients' perspectives on clinical practices for alleviating distress and promoting empowerment during awake craniotomies. Br J Neurosurg. 2021;0(0):1–12. https://doi.org/10.1080/02688697.2021.2005773.
56. Hejrati N, Spieler D, Samuel R, Regli L, Weyerbrock A, Surbeck W. Conscious experience and psychological consequences of awake craniotomy. World Neurosurg. 2019;129:e381–6. https://doi.org/10.1016/j.wneu.2019.05.156.
57. Starowicz-Filip A, Prochwicz K, Myszka A, et al. Subjective experience, cognitive functioning and trauma level of patients undergoing awake craniotomy due to brain tumor—preliminary study. Appl Neuropsychol. 2020;0(0):1–10. https://doi.org/10.1080/23279095.2020.1831500.
58. Klimek M, van der Horst PH, Hoeks SE, Stolker RJ. Quality and quantity of memories in patients who undergo awake brain tumor resection. World Neurosurg. 2018;109:e258–64. https://doi.org/10.1016/j.wneu.2017.09.158.
59. Potters JW, Klimek M. Awake craniotomy: improving the patient's experience. Curr Opin Anaesthesiol.

2015;28(5):511–6. https://doi.org/10.1097/ACO.0000000000000231.
60. Aabedi A, Ahn E, Kakaizada S, et al. Assessment of wakefulness during awake craniotomy to predict intraoperative language performance. J Neurosurg. 2020;132(6):1930–7. https://doi.org/10.3171/2F2019.2.JNS183486.
61. Papatzalas C, Fountas K, Kapsalaki E, Papathanasiou I. The use of standardized intraoperative language tests in awake craniotomies: a scoping review. Cham: Springer; 2021. https://doi.org/10.1007/s11065-021-09492-6.
62. Suarez-meade P, Marenco-hillembrand L, Prevatt C, et al. Awake vs. asleep motor mapping for glioma resection: a systematic review and meta-analysis. Acta Neurochir. 2020;162:1709. https://doi.org/10.1007/s00701-020-04357-y.
63. De Witte E, Satoer D, Colle H, Robert E, Visch-Brink E, Mariën P. Subcortical language and non-language mapping in awake brain surgery: the use of multimodal tests. Acta Neurochir. 2015;157(4):577–88. https://doi.org/10.1007/s00701-014-2317-0.
64. Verst SM, de Castro I, Scappini-Junior W, et al. Methodology for creating and validating object naming and semantic tests used by Verst-Maldaun language assessment during awake craniotomies. Clin Neurol Neurosurg. 2021;202(November 2020):3–10. https://doi.org/10.1016/j.clineuro.2021.106485.
65. Duffau H. Awake surgery for left posterior insular low-grade glioma through the parietorolandic operculum: the need to preserve the functional connectivity. A case series. Front Surg. 2022;8(January):1–8. https://doi.org/10.3389/fsurg.2021.824003.
66. Boetto J, Bertram L, Moulinié G, Herbet G, Moritz-Gasser S, Duffau H. Electrocorticography is not necessary during awake brain surgery for gliomas. World Neurosurg. 2016;91:656–7. https://doi.org/10.1016/j.wneu.2016.03.030.
67. Mahboob S, McPhillips R, Qiu Z, et al. Intraoperative ultrasound-guided resection of gliomas: a meta-analysis and review of the literature. World Neurosurg. 2016;92:255–63. https://doi.org/10.1016/j.wneu.2016.05.007.
68. Sweeney JF, Smith H, Taplin AL, Perloff E, Adamo MA. Effcacy of intraoperative ultrasonography in neurosurgical tumor resection. J Neurosurg Pediatr. 2018;21(5):504–10. https://doi.org/10.3171/2017.11.PEDS17473.
69. Duffau H. Lessons from brain mapping in surgery for low-grade glioma: insights into associations between tumour and brain plasticity. Lancet Neurol. 2005;4(8):476–86. https://doi.org/10.1016/S1474-4422(05)70140-X.
70. Michaud K, Duffau H. Surgery of insular and paralimbic diffuse low-grade gliomas: technical considerations. J Neuro-Oncol. 2016;130(2):289–98. https://doi.org/10.1007/s11060-016-2120-2.
71. Duffau H, Capelle L, Denvil D, et al. Usefulness of intraoperative electrical subcortical mapping during surgery for low-grade gliomas located within eloquent brain regions: functional results in a consecutive series of 103 patients. J Neurosurg. 2003;98(4):764–78. https://doi.org/10.3171/jns.2003.98.4.0764.
72. Duffau H, Moritz-Gasser S, Gatignol P. Functional outcome after language mapping for insular World Health Organization grade II gliomas in the dominant hemisphere: experience with 24 patients. Neurosurg Focus. 2009;27(2):1–10. https://doi.org/10.3171/2009.5.FOCUS0938.
73. Young JS, Lee AT, Chang EF. A review of cortical and subcortical stimulation mapping for language. Neurosurgery. 2021;89(3):331–42. https://doi.org/10.1093/neuros/nyaa436.
74. Lemaitre A, Herbet G, Ng S, Moritz-gasser S, Duffau H. Cognitive preservation following awake mapping-based neurosurgery for low-grade gliomas: a longitudinal, within-patient design study. Neuro Oncol. 2021;24(November):1–13.
75. Duffau H. New philosophy, clinical pearls, and methods for intraoperative cognition mapping and monitoring "à la carte" in brain tumor patients. Neurosurgery. 2021;88(5):919–30. https://doi.org/10.1093/neuros/nyaa363.
76. Duffau H. Updated perspectives on awake neurosurgery with cognitive and emotional assessment for patients with low-grade gliomas. Expert Rev Neurother. 2021;21(4):463–73. https://doi.org/10.1080/14737175.2021.1901583.
77. Surbeck W, Hildebrandt G, Duffau H. The evolution of brain surgery on awake patients. Acta Neurochir. 2015;157(1):77–84. https://doi.org/10.1007/s00701-014-2249-8.
78. Wang YC, Lee CC, Takami H, et al. Awake craniotomies for epileptic gliomas: intraoperative and postoperative seizure control and prognostic factors. J Neuro-Oncol. 2019;142(3):577–86. https://doi.org/10.1007/s11060-019-03131-0.
79. Nossek E, Matot I, Shahar T, et al. Intraoperative seizures during awake craniotomy: incidence and consequences: analysis of 477 patients. Neurosurgery. 2013;73(1):135–40. https://doi.org/10.1227/01.neu.0000429847.91707.97.
80. Cochereau J, Herbet G, Duffau H. Patients with incidental WHO grade II glioma frequently suffer from neuropsychological disturbances. Acta Neurochir. 2016;158(2):305–12. https://doi.org/10.1007/s00701-015-2674-3.
81. Chan-Seng E, Moritz-Gasser S, Duffau H. Awake mapping for low-grade gliomas involving the left sagittal stratum: anatomofunctional and surgical considerations: clinical article. J Neurosurg. 2014;120(5):1069–77. https://doi.org/10.3171/2014.1.JNS132015.
82. Still MEH, Roux A, Huberfeld G, et al. Extent of resection and residual tumor thresholds for postoperative total seizure freedom in epileptic adult patients harboring a supratentorial diffuse low-grade glioma. Neurosurgery. 2019;85(2):E332–9. https://doi.org/10.1093/neuros/nyy481.

83. Fang S, Zhou C, Wang L, et al. Characteristic alterations of network in patients with intraoperative stimulation-induced seizures during awake craniotomy. Front Neurol. 2021;12(March):1–10. https://doi.org/10.3389/fneur.2021.602716.
84. Roca E, Pallud J, Guerrini F, Panciani PP, Fontanella M, Spena G. Stimulation-related intraoperative seizures during awake surgery: a review of available evidences. Neurosurg Rev. 2020;43(1):87–93. https://doi.org/10.1007/s10143-019-01214-0.
85. Spena G, Roca E, Guerrini F, et al. Risk factors for intraoperative stimulation-related seizures during awake surgery: an analysis of 109 consecutive patients. J Neuro-Oncol. 2019;145(2):295–300. https://doi.org/10.1007/s11060-019-03295-9.
86. Otani R, Yamada R, Kawaguchi K, Kikuchi M, Kushihara Y, Shinoura N. Utility of monitoring the serum levetiracetam concentration for intraoperative seizure control during awake craniotomy. J Clin Neurosci. 2021;89:279–82. https://doi.org/10.1016/j.jocn.2021.05.028.
87. Ng S, Lemaitre A-L, Moritz-Gasser S, Herbet G, Duffau H. Recurrent low-grade gliomas: does reoperation affect neurocognitive functioning? Neurosurgery. 2021;90(2):221–32. https://doi.org/10.1227/neu.0000000000001784.
88. Bunyaratavej K, Sangtongjaraskul S, Lerdsirisopon S, Tuchinda L. Continuous physical examination during subcortical resection in awake craniotomy patients: its usefulness and surgical outcome. Clin Neurol Neurosurg. 2016;147:34. https://doi.org/10.1016/j.clineuro.2016.05.021.
89. Alimohamadi M, Shirani M, Shariat-moharreri R, et al. Application of awake craniotomy and intraoperative brain mapping for surgical resection of insular gliomas of the dominant hemisphere. World Neurosurg. 2016;92:151–8. https://doi.org/10.1016/j.wneu.2016.04.079.
90. Mansur A, Oswari S, Octavian P, Wahjoepramono P, Kusdiansah M, Bernstein M. Awake craniotomy in a low- to middle-income country: a sustainability analysis. World Neurosurg. 2018;118:332–41. https://doi.org/10.1016/j.wneu.2018.07.149.
91. Nossek E, Matot I, Shahar T, et al. Failed awake craniotomy: a retrospective analysis in 424 patients undergoing craniotomy for brain tumor; clinical article. J Neurosurg. 2013;118(2):243–9. https://doi.org/10.3171/2012.10.JNS12511.
92. Stevanovic A, Rossaint R, Veldeman M, Bilotta F. Anaesthesia management for awake craniotomy: systematic review and meta-analysis. PLoS One. 2016;11(5):12–23. https://doi.org/10.1371/journal.pone.0156448.
93. Balki M, Manninen PH, Mcguire GP, El-beheiry H, Bernstein M. Venous air embolism during awake craniotomy in a supine patient. Can J Anesth. 2003;50:835–8.
94. Abaziou T, Tincres F, Mrozek S, et al. Incidence and predicting factors of perioperative complications during monitored anesthesia care for awake craniotomy. J Clin Anesth. 2020;64(April):109811. https://doi.org/10.1016/j.jclinane.2020.109811.
95. Khu KJ, Doglietto F, Radovanovic I, et al. Patients' perceptions of awake and outpatient craniotomy for brain tumor: a qualitative study—clinical article. J Neurosurg. 2010;112(5):1056–60. https://doi.org/10.3171/2009.6.JNS09716.
96. Palese A, Skrap M, Fachin M, Visioli S, Zannini L. The experience of patients undergoing awake craniotomy: in the patients' own words. A qualitative study. Cancer Nurs. 2008;31(2):166–72. https://doi.org/10.1097/01.NCC.0000305699.97625.dc.
97. Trimble G, McStravick C, Farling P, et al. Awake craniotomy for glioma resection: technical aspects and initial results in a single institution. Br J Neurosurg. 2015;29(6):836–42. https://doi.org/10.3109/02688697.2015.1054354.
98. Jose GRB, Legaspi GD. Challenges in the performance of awake craniotomies in the Philippine general hospital: a case series. Acta Med Philipp. 2021;56:1–11. https://doi.org/10.47895/amp.vi0.1738.

Post Awake Craniotomy Care <Postoperative Care, Pain, Seizures, Postoperative Nausea and Vomiting>

Roger M. Krzyzewski
and Lucas Alverne Freitas Albuquerque

1 Introduction

During the postoperative period, patients are prone to complications after brain tumor surgery and frequency can occur up to 68% [1]. Major complications are new sensorimotor deficits which include transient and permanent, new language deficit, postoperative nausea, vomiting, decreased consciousness, postoperative seizures, and postoperative pain. However, new language deficit (up to 40% with only 4% remaining permanent) occurs most often [1]. Despite relatively high frequency of postoperative adverse events most of them are transient and subside during the same hospitalization. In comparison to the general anesthesia (GA), awake craniotomy for glioblastoma cases carries much lower risk for postoperative complications [2].

Some studies postulate same-day discharge after awake craniotomy. This requires identifying patients who might need additional attention during the postoperative period. For example, in a retrospective review of 424 cases, 137 patients were discharged on postoperative day one. Most of these patients were male, had right-sided tumors, fewer coexisting medical conditions, lower modified Rankin Scale score, smaller maximal lesions diameter, supratentorial lesions and no need for intubation or lumbar drainage implying that further attention was not indicated [3].

The quality of postoperative care can determine the risk of readmission occurring up to 6%. Neurological decline and seizures are the leading cause for readmissions [4]. Redo surgery and patients with identified intraoperative hemorrhage were also associated with readmission. Patients undergoing surgery for recurrent tumors and patients that had hemorrhagic complications during surgery should receive focused attention postoperatively. It is interesting that age, malignancy, and preoperative functional status were not associated with readmission [4].

Immediate motor deficit occurs in up to 38% of patients and 13% of them remain without improvement after 3 months [5]. After awake craniotomy, new neurological deficits are independently associated with subcortical resection and significant Diffusion Weighted Imaging (DWI) changes on MRI [5].

Failed awake craniotomy (awake craniotomy converted to GA) can predict most serious complications during postoperative care (up to 6.4%) and is associated with postoperative complications such as hemorrhage or cardiovascular events. Most common causes of failed awake cra-

R. M. Krzyzewski (✉)
Department of Neurosurgery and Neurotraumatology, Jagiellonian University Medical College, Kraków, Poland
e-mail: roger.krzyzewski@uj.edu.pl

L. A. F. Albuquerque
Department of Neurosurgery, General Hospital of Fortaleza, Fortaleza, Ceará, Brazil

A. Pour-Rashidi, J. Aarabi (eds.), *The Principles of Successful Awake Craniotomy*,
https://doi.org/10.1007/978-981-99-2985-6_8

2.4 Antiepileptic Drugs

The most widely used antiepileptic drugs in treatment for pain are gabapentin and α2δ ligands which are derivatives of the inhibitory neurotransmitter gamma-aminobutyric acid (GABA) [33] Perioperative administration of gabapentin in patients undergoing scheduled craniotomy showed great results in diminishing postoperative pain within 24 h but its effects were similar to the non-gabapentin group after 48 h. Moreover, gabapentin administration produced lower incidence of vomiting but did not decrease the frequency of nausea [34], and it should be administered slowly and in divided doses. The maximum dosage is 3600 mg given orally should be achieved between 7–10 days [33]. If high doses of gabapentin are given rapidly it can produce vertigo, confusion, nausea, and vomiting. A Proposed protocol for administration of gabapentin in patients undergoing craniotomy is 600 mg of gabapentin given orally the night prior to surgery and another 600 mg dosage 2 h prior to induction of anesthesia [34]. Another protocol suggests administration of 4 mg dexamethasone together with two dosages of 600 mg of gabapentin that produces better effects in terms of controlling postoperative nausea and vomiting with no effect on postoperative pain or opioid consumption [35]. Of note, preoperative gabapentin diminished the need for intraoperative propofol and remifentanil but did not influence postoperative opioid consumption [34].

Pregabalin is a gabapentinoid with a distinct pharmacological profile that is preferable for patients with craniotomy, awake craniotomy, and other neurosurgical interventions. The pharmacodynamics of gabapentin are less predictable because gabapentin concentration increases nonlinearly and doses which are given orally cannot measure plasma levels of gabapentin. Pregabalin in absorbed more rapidly, and its plasma concentration is proportionate to an oral dose. Pregabalin is slightly more effective in neuropathic pain but has significantly stronger anti-epileptic effects [36]. Pregabalin is preferable in patients with preexisting epilepsy and neuropathic pain could benefit more from pregabalin in perioperative period. A randomized, double-blinded, placebo-controlled study examined the effects of a single dose of 150 mg of pregabalin before surgery and 150 mg of pregabalin twice daily within 72 h post-surgery in neurosurgical patients [37]. The study found that this protocol significantly reduced presurgical anxiety. This intervention yielded better pain score, better pain control, and reduced consumption of antiemetics and analgesics. Moreover, there were no adverse events associated with the administration of pregabalin [37]. Another randomized control study examined administration of 75 mg and 150 mg of pregabalin orally prior to induction of anesthesia in comparison to placebo. This study found that there were no differences in pain levels between 75 and 150 mg, but the group receiving 150 mg required less fentanyl in the postoperative period [38].

Pregabalin is an effective drug in the treatment of preoperative anxiety, improving preoperative sleep, limiting pain and opioid use, but only at a dose of at least 150 mg. It can be given as little as 1.5 h prior to surgery to produce results and can be continued up to 72 h after surgery to produce robust effects in the treatment of postoperative pain. There are no studies addressing the use of pregabalin specifically in terms of awake craniotomy. One might hypothesize that pregabalin could reduce preoperative anxiety associated with awake craniotomy; therefore, it might be preferred in preparation for awake craniotomy in addition to providing better sleep. It has been shown that in awake vitro-retinal surgery, patients premedicated with pregabalin showed higher cooperation than placebo-controlled and needed lower doses of benzodiazepine [39].

2.5 Opioid Analgesia

Intraoperative analgesia is usually administered by remifentanil or fentanyl, and opioids are given for postoperative analgesia that are safe and effective along with agents that do not depress respiration. Sudheer et al. [40] found that morphine produced better analgesic effects after craniotomy in comparison to tramadol and codeine. In those patients, nausea and vomiting was present in 50% of those receiving tramadol, but only in 20% receiving morphine and 29% receiving codeine. There is some evidence that titrated morphine can be safely used after craniotomy in both adults and children [41].

The benefit of using tramadol in awake craniotomy is controversial due to higher risk of epileptic seizures. A large cohort study of nearly 10,000 patients using tramadol showed that 80 of them had their first epileptic seizure after tramadol use [42]. After adjusting for confounding variables, they found that the use of tramadol increased the risk of seizure by two to six folds. Risk factors for seizure after tramadol use are ages 25–54 years, history of alcohol abuse, stroke, and head injury. Patients receiving higher doses of tramadol had a higher risk of seizures [42]. Awake craniotomy carries a greater risk of injury due to epileptic seizures than craniotomy under GA, and all epileptogenic agents should be avoided.

In terms of treatment of postoperative pain after awake craniotomy, one study compared non-opioid analgesia with paracetamol only. This was a combination of paracetamol with tramadol, compared to paracetamol and nalbuphine. Patients that received nalbuphine (a strong derivative of morphine) reported significantly lower pain and required fewer infusions of analgesics. Moreover, patients receiving nalbuphine instead of tramadol had significantly lower incidences of postoperative nausea and vomiting [43]. Paracetamol alone is not suitable for treatment of pain after awake craniotomy [43].

Despite ERAS protocol suggesting that all opioids should be avoided to provide better functional outcome after surgery, a recent patient-controlled remifentanil administration system was proposed as a safe and effective method of pain treatment after awake craniotomy [44]. Morphine and other strong opioids still remain superior to a non-opioid analgesia with dexmedetomidine scalp block in terms of postoperative pain control [45].

2.6 Sumatriptan

An emerging concept in the treatment of postoperative pain after craniotomy is the introduction of subcutaneous sumatriptan which is a selective serotonin receptor agonist primarily used in the treatment of migraine and other primary headaches [46]. Subcutaneous sumatriptan has been described to significantly reduce pain and need for opioids used in both adults and children after craniotomy [46]. The results of a randomized, double-blinded, placebo-controlled subcutaneous sumatriptan study for the treatment of post-craniotomy pain (SUPS trial) are yet to be published [47]. Sumatriptan has been confirmed by a randomized controlled trial to improve headache and quality of outcome after cranial nerve decompression [48].

3 Postoperative Nausea and Vomiting

Cumulative risk for postoperative nausea and vomiting after supratentorial craniotomy varies between 50 and 70% [49]. Infratentorial surgery carries a much greater risk for postoperative nausea, and vomiting [50]. Postoperative nausea and vomiting may lead to aspiration, increased intracranial pressure, postoperative epileptic seizure, intracranial bleeding, and new neurological deficits.

There is no association between tumor malignancy surgery with awake craniotomy and incidence of postoperative nausea and vomiting [51]. In contrast, this study suggested that there was lack of association between tumor malignancy and postoperative nausea and vomiting in significantly younger aged patients with low-grade tumors.

When comparing awake surgery to GA in patients undergoing awake craniotomy, there were significantly fewer episodes of nausea and vomiting reported and less need for antiemetic drugs [52]. This effect remained significant up to 4 h after surgery. Only 4% of patients complained of nausea and none of them experienced vomiting. In comparison within the first 4 h, up to 23% of patients after GA had nausea and 11% found

7 Conclusion

In the postoperative period, the main issues that should be addressed are pain, nausea, and vomiting, seizure activity, hypothermia, anxiety, and any new neurological deficits. Postoperative pain can be relieved by administering paracetamol at a maximum dose of 4 g daily and metamizole at 5 g daily combined with NSAIDs. There is emerging evidence that NSAIDS such as diclofenac (100 mg) or dexketoprofen (50 mg) provide better pain control with little influence on clotting or platelet function. Dexketoprofen and metamizole can decrease consumption of opioids. Flupirinte can be incorporated especially after awake procedure to decrease pain and anxiety. Gabapentinoids are safe and effective in treatment of postoperative pain, nausea, vomiting, and anxiety both prior to and after craniotomy. Gabapentin 600 mg orally should be introduced the night before surgery and 600 mg 2 h prior to induction of anesthesia. Pregabalin produces more robust results than gabapentin, but it should be given in divided doses of at least 150 mg to produce effects other than anxiolytics and hypnotics. When given at a dose of 150 mg on the night prior to surgery and 1.5 h prior to induction of anesthesia, it can reduce pain, decrease incidence of nausea and vomiting, limit the need for opioids, and reduce anxiety. Implementation of dexmedetomidine during the procedure greatly enhances the quality of postoperative course of treatment. Tramadol and codeine should be a second choice as opioid analgesics after awake craniotomy due to a slightly less favorable pharmacological profile and emetogenic properties. Moreover, tramadol might have slight epileptogenic properties which is important in neurosurgical procedures. Strong opioids such as morphine and oxycodone should be used sparingly but are safe. Principles of ERAS protocol postulate a growing role of non-opioid analgesia. Subcutaneous sumatriptan seems to produce good results after craniotomy and deserves attention.

Up to 70% of patients after elective craniotomy suffer from nausea and vomiting. During post-awake craniotomy patients have a significantly lower incidence of nausea and vomiting within the first 4 h, but the same risk as posterior fossa procedures after 4 h. A single dose of dexamethasone prior to awake craniotomy for brain tumor can significantly reduce frequency of vomiting in the postoperative period. The most effective drug treatment for postoperative nausea and vomiting are dexamethasone and serotonin antagonists. Also, there is growing evidence for use of gabapentin. There is low-quality evidence that scopolamine and aprepitant might have some use. Serotonin antagonists might be less effective in pediatric patients.

Postoperative seizures are particularly associated with awake craniotomy due to direct electrical stimulation of the brain during surgery that can produce seizures both during and after surgery. There is still lack of convincing evidence in favor of any particular agent. Most commonly used agents are phenytoin, phenobarbital, carbamazepine, and lamotrigine. Moreover, there are still no supporting data about the benefits of prophylactic anti-seizure medication in awake craniotomy. Retrospective studies lean toward prophylactic use of lamotrigine prior to and phenytoin after surgery. Patients particularly with epileptogenic lesions or a history of epilepsy prior to the surgery should receive antiepileptic drugs prior to surgery and then be considered for routine dual therapy. Patients that experienced epileptic seizures during surgery are at risk for developing seizures postoperatively and at greater risk of readmission overall.

References

1. Kwinta BM, Myszka AM, Bigaj MM, Krzyżewski RM, Starowicz-Filip A. Intra- and postoperative adverse events in awake craniotomy for intrinsic supratentorial brain tumors. Neurol Sci. 2021;42:1437–41.
2. Gerritsen JKW, Viëtor CL, Rizopoulos D, Schouten JW, Klimek M, Dirven CMF, Vincent AJPE. Awake craniotomy versus craniotomy under general anesthesia without surgery adjuncts for supratentorial glioblastoma in eloquent areas: a retrospective matched case-control study. Acta Neurochir. 2019;161:307–15.
3. Richardson AM, McCarthy DJ, Sandhu J, Mayrand R, Guerrero C, Rosenberg C, Gernsback JE, Komotar R,

Ivan M. Predictors of successful discharge of patients on postoperative day 1 after craniotomy for brain tumor. World Neurosurg. 2019;126:e869–77.
4. Takami H, Venkatraghavan L, Bernstein M. Perioperative factors affecting readmission after awake craniotomy: analysis of 609 consecutive cases. World Neurosurg. 2021;134:1631. https://doi.org/10.1016/J.WNEU.2021.11.010.
5. Trinh VT, Fahim DK, Shah K, Tummala S, McCutcheon IE, Sawaya R, Suki D, Prabhu SS. Subcortical injury is an independent predictor of worsening neurological deficits following awake craniotomy procedures. Neurosurgery. 2013;72:160–9.
6. Nossek E, Matot I, Shahar T, Barzilai O, Rapoport Y, Gonen T, Sela G, Korn A, Hayat D, Ram Z. Failed awake craniotomy: a retrospective analysis in 424 patients undergoing craniotomy for brain tumor. J Neurosurg. 2013;118:243–9.
7. Ljungqvist O, Scott M, Fearon KC. Enhanced recovery after surgery: a review. JAMA Surg. 2017;152:292–8.
8. Hagan KB, Bhavsar S, Raza SM, et al. Enhanced recovery after surgery for oncological craniotomies. J Clin Neurosci. 2016;24:10–6.
9. Wang L, Cai H, Wang Y, Liu J, Chen T, Liu J, Huang J, Guo Q, Zou W. Enhanced recovery after elective craniotomy: a randomized controlled trial. J Clin Anesth. 2022;76:110575. https://doi.org/10.1016/J.JCLINANE.2021.110575.
10. Jun CY, Nie C, Lu H, Zhang L, Lin CH, Yong WS, Li W, Shen S, Wang H. Monitored anesthetic care combined with scalp nerve block in awake craniotomy: an effective attempt at enhanced recovery after neurosurgery. World Neurosurg. 2021;154:e509–19.
11. Bojaxhi E, Louie C, ReFaey K, Gruenbaum SE, Leone BJ, Bechtel P, Barbosa MP, Chaichana KL, Quinones-Hinojosa A. Reduced pain and opioid use in the early postoperative period in patients undergoing a frontotemporal craniotomy under regional vs general anesthesia. World Neurosurg. 2021;150:e31–7.
12. Eseonu CI, Rincon-Torroella J, ReFaey K, Lee YM, Nangiana J, Vivas-Buitrago T, Quiñones-Hinojosa A. Awake craniotomy vs craniotomy under general anesthesia for perirolandic gliomas: evaluating perioperative complications and extent of resection. Neurosurgery. 2017;81:481–9.
13. Mordhorst C, Latz B, Kerz T, Wisser G, Schmidt A, Schneider A, Jahn-Eimermacher A, Werner C, Engelhard K. Prospective assessment of postoperative pain after craniotomy. J Neurosurg Anesthesiol. 2010;22:202–6.
14. Thibault M, Girard F, Moumdjian R, Chouinard P, Boudreault D, Ruel M. Craniotomy site influences postoperative pain following neurosurgical procedures: a retrospective study. Can J Anaesth. 2007;54:544–8.
15. Bronco A, Pietrini D, Lamperti M, et al. Incidence of pain after craniotomy in children. Paediatr Anaesth. 2014;24:781–7.
16. Bala I, Gupta B, Vhardwaj N, Ghai B, Khosla VK. Effect of scalp block on postoperative pain relief in craniotomy patients. Anaesth Intensive Care. 2006;34:224–7.
17. Guilfoyle MR, Helmy A, Duane D, Hutchinson PJA. Regional scalp block for postcraniotomy analgesia: a systematic review and meta-analysis. Anesth Analg. 2013;116:1093–102.
18. Ayoub C, Girard F, Boudreault D, Chouinard P, Ruel M, Moumdjian R. A comparison between scalp nerve block and morphine for transitional analgesia after remifentanil-based anesthesia in neurosurgery. Anesth Analg. 2006;103:1237–40.
19. Costello TG, Cormack JR, Mather LE, LaFerlita B, Murphy MA, Harris K. Plasma levobupivacaine concentrations following scalp block in patients undergoing awake craniotomy. Br J Anaesth. 2005;94:848–51.
20. Nguyen A, Girard F, Boudreault D, Fugère F, Ruel M, Moumdjian R, Bouthilier A, Caron JL, Bojanowski MW, Girard DC. Scalp nerve blocks decrease the severity of pain after craniotomy. Anesth Analg. 2001;93:1272–6.
21. Akhigbe T, Zolnourian A. Use of regional scalp block for pain management after craniotomy: review of literature and critical appraisal of evidence. J Clin Neurosci. 2017;45:44–7.
22. Song J, Ji Q, Sun Q, Gao T, Liu K, Li L. The opioid-sparing effect of intraoperative dexmedetomidine infusion after craniotomy. J Neurosurg Anesthesiol. 2016;28:14–20.
23. Sivakumar W, Jensen M, Martinez J, Tanana M, Duncan N, Hoesch R, Riva-Cambrin JK, Kilburg C, Ansari S, House PA. Intravenous acetaminophen for postoperative supratentorial craniotomy pain: a prospective, randomized, double-blinded, placebo-controlled trial. J Neurosurg. 2018;130:766–72.
24. Artime CA, Aijazi H, Zhang H, Syed T, Cai C, Gumbert SD, Ferrario L, Normand KC, Williams GW, Hagberg CA. Scheduled intravenous acetaminophen improves patient satisfaction with Postcraniotomy pain management: a prospective, randomized, placebo-controlled, double-blind study. J Neurosurg Anesthesiol. 2018;30:231–6.
25. Ebada MA, Ali AS, Elshakankiry A, et al. Should intravenous acetaminophen be considered for post craniotomy pain management? A meta-analysis of randomized controlled trials. J Neurosurg Sci. 2021;66:413–9. https://doi.org/10.23736/S0390-5616.21.05402-3.
26. Rahimi SY, Vender JR, Macomson SD, French A, Smith JR, Alleyne CH. Postoperative pain management after craniotomy: evaluation and cost analysis. Neurosurgery. 2006;59:852–7.
27. Williams DL, Pemberton E, Leslie K. Effect of intravenous parecoxib on post-craniotomy pain. Br J Anaesth. 2011;107:398–403.
28. Rajkiran R, Lal Soni S, Jangra K, Bhagat H, Singh A, Singh A, Panda NB, Kaloria N. Diclofenac is superior to paracetamol in postoperative pain scores and analgesic consumption in supratentorial craniotomy with no difference in platelet and clot function: a prospective randomized controlled trial. J

Neurosurg Anesthesiol. 2021;34(3):321–6. https://doi.org/10.1097/ANA.0000000000000765.
29. Grossman R, Ram Z, Perel A, Yusim Y, Zaslansky R, Berkenstadt H. Control of postoperative pain after awake craniotomy with local intradermal analgesia and metamizol. Isr Med Assoc J. 2007;9:380–2.
30. Dilmen OK, Akcil EF, Tunali Y, Karabulut ES, Bahar M, Altindas F, Vehid H, Yentur E. Postoperative analgesia for supratentorial craniotomy. Clin Neurol Neurosurg. 2016;146:90–5.
31. Yadav G, Choupoo S, Das SK, Das SK, Behera SS, Khuba S, Mishra LD, Singh DK. Evaluating the role of flupirtine for postcraniotomy pain and compare it with diclofenac sodium: a prospective, randomized, double blind, placebo-controlled study. J Neurosurg Anesthesiol. 2014;26:32–6.
32. Yadav G, Jain G, Singh M. Role of flupirtine in reducing preoperative anxiety of patients undergoing craniotomy procedure. Saudi J Anaesth. 2017;11:158–62.
33. Calandre EP, Rico-Villademoros F, Slim M. Alpha2delta ligands, gabapentin, pregabalin and mirogabalin: a review of their clinical pharmacology and therapeutic use. Expert Rev Neurother. 2016;16:1263–77. https://doi.org/10.1080/14737175 20161202764.
34. Zeng M, Dong J, Lin N, Zhang W, Zhang K, Peng K, Wang D, Zhao Y, Peng Y, Han R. Preoperative gabapentin administration improves acute postoperative analgesia in patients undergoing craniotomy: a randomized controlled trial. J Neurosurg Anesthesiol. 2019;31:392–8.
35. Misra S, Parthasarathi G, Vilanilam GC. The effect of gabapentin premedication on postoperative nausea, vomiting, and pain in patients on preoperative dexamethasone undergoing craniotomy for intracranial tumors. J Neurosurg Anesthesiol. 2013;25:386–91.
36. Bockbrader HN, Wesche D, Miller R, Chapel S, Janiczek N, Burger P. A comparison of the pharmacokinetics and pharmacodynamics of pregabalin and gabapentin. Clin Pharmacokinet. 2012;49(10):661–9.
37. Shimony N, Amit U, Minz B, Grossman R, Dany MA, Gonen L, Kandov K, Ram Z, Weinbroum AA. Perioperative pregabalin for reducing pain, analgesic consumption, and anxiety and enhancing sleep quality in elective neurosurgical patients: a prospective, randomized, double-blind, and controlled clinical study. J Neurosurg. 2016;125:1513–22.
38. Lamsal R, Mahajan C, Chauhan V, Gupta N, Mishra N, Rath GP. Effect of pregabalin on postcraniotomy pain in patients undergoing supratentorial tumor surgery: a randomized, double-blind, placebo-controlled trial. J Neurosci Rural Pract. 2019;10:641.
39. Elrashidy A, Khattab AM, Elseify ZA, Oriby ME. Perioperative anxiolytic and analgesic effects of Pregabalin in Vitreo-retinal surgery: a randomized, double-blind study. Anesth Pain Med. 2021;11(4):e117414. https://doi.org/10.5812/AAPM.117414.
40. Sudheer PS, Logan SW, Terblanche C, Ateleanu B, Hall JE. Comparison of the analgesic efficacy and respiratory effects of morphine, tramadol and codeine after craniotomy. Anaesthesia. 2007;62:555–60.
41. Warren DT, Bowen-Roberts T, Ou C, Purdy R, Steinbok P. Safety and efficacy of continuous morphine infusions following pediatric cranial surgery in a surgical ward setting. Childs Nerv Syst. 2010;26:1535–41.
42. Gardner JS, Blough D, Drinkard CR, Shatin D, Anderson G, Graham D, Alderfer R. Tramadol and seizures: a surveillance study in a managed care population. Pharmacotherapy. 2000;20:1423–31.
43. Verchère E, Grenier B, Mesli A, Siao D, Sesay M, Maurette P. Postoperative pain management after supratentorial craniotomy. J Neurosurg Anesthesiol. 2002;14:96–101.
44. Ijaz MK, Moore M. Remifentanil patient-controlled analgesia in awake craniotomy: an introduction of an innovative technique. J Neurosurg Anesthesiol. 2020;32:367.
45. Darmawikarta D, Sourour M, Couban R, Kamath S, Reddy KKV, Shanthanna H. Opioid-free analgesia for supratentorial craniotomies: a systematic review. Can J Neurol Sci. 2019;46:415–22.
46. Patel KS, Laiwalla AN, DiCesare JAT, Garrett MC, Wang AC. Subcutaneous sumatriptan: association with decreases in postoperative pain and opioid use after elective cranial surgery. J Neurosurg. 2020;134:401–9.
47. Licina A, Russell J, Silvers A, Jin X, Denny J. Subcutaneous sumatriptan for the treatment of postcraniotomy pain (SUPS trial): protocol for a randomised double-blinded placebo controlled trial. BMJ Open. 2019;9:e032388. https://doi.org/10.1136/BMJOPEN-2019-032388.
48. Venkatraghavan L, Li L, Bailey T, Manninen PH, Tymianski M. Sumatriptan improves postoperative quality of recovery and reduces postcraniotomy headache after cranial nerve decompression. Br J Anaesth. 2016;117:73–9.
49. Fabling JM, Gan TJ, El-Moalem HE, Warner DS, Borel CO. A randomized, double-blinded comparison of ondansetron, droperidol, and placebo for prevention of postoperative nausea and vomiting after supratentorial craniotomy. Anesth Analg. 2000;91:358–61.
50. Fabling JM, Gan TJ, Guy J, Borel CO, El-Moalem HE, Warner DS. Postoperative nausea and vomiting: a retrospective analysis. J Neurosurg Anesthesiol. 1997;9(4):308–12. https://journals.lww.com/jnsa/Abstract/1997/10000/Postoperative_Nausea_and_Vomiting__A_Retrospective.3.aspx. Accessed 1 Feb 2022.
51. Ouyang MW, McDonagh DL, Phillips-Bute B, James ML, Friedman AH, Gan TJ. Comparison of postoperative nausea between benign and malignant brain tumor patients undergoing awake craniotomy: a retrospective analysis. Curr Med Res Opin. 2013;29:1039–44.
52. Manninen PH, Tan TK. Postoperative nausea and vomiting after craniotomy for tumor surgery: a comparison between awake craniotomy and general anesthesia. J Clin Anesth. 2002;14:279–83.

53. Kamata K, Morioka N, Maruyama T, Komayama N, Nitta M, Muragaki Y, Kawamata T, Ozaki M. The effect of single low-dose dexamethasone on vomiting during awake craniotomy. J Anesth. 2016;30:941–8.
54. Jain V, Mitra JK, Rath GP, Prabhakar H, Bithal PK, Dash HH. A randomized, double-blinded comparison of ondansetron, granisetron, and placebo for prevention of postoperative nausea and vomiting after supratentorial craniotomy. J Neurosurg Anesthesiol. 2009;21:226–30.
55. Knape JTA, Adriaensen H, Van Aken H, Blunnie WP, Carlsson C, Dupont M, Pasch T. Scheduled prophylactic ondansetron administration did not improve its antiemetic efficacy after intracranial tumour resection surgery in children. Eur J Anaesthesiol. 2007;24:563–7.
56. Lee A, Chan SKC, Fan LTY. Stimulation of the wrist acupuncture point PC6 for preventing postoperative nausea and vomiting. Cochrane Database Syst Rev. 2015;2016:CD003281. https://doi.org/10.1002/14651858.CD003281.PUB4.
57. Kahlenberg CA, Fadul CE, Roberts DW, Thadani VM, Bujarski KA, Scott RC, Jobst BC. Seizure prognosis of patients with low-grade tumors. Seizure. 2012;21:540–5.
58. Dewan MC, White-Dzuro GA, Brinson PR, Thompson RC, Chambless LB. Perioperative seizure in patients with glioma is associated with longer hospitalization, higher readmission, and decreased overall survival. J Neurosurg. 2016;125:1033–41.
59. Klimek M, Dammers R. Antiepileptic drug therapy in the perioperative course of neurosurgical patients. Curr Opin Anaesthesiol. 2010;23:564–7.
60. Gonen T, Grossman R, Sitt R, Nossek E, Yanaki R, Cagnano E, Korn A, Hayat D, Ram Z. Tumor location and IDH1 mutation may predict intraoperative seizures during awake craniotomy. J Neurosurg. 2014;121:1133–8.
61. Greenhalgh J, Weston J, Dundar Y, Nevitt SJ, Marson AG. Antiepileptic drugs as prophylaxis for postcraniotomy seizures. Cochrane Database Syst Rev. 2020;4:CD007286. https://doi.org/10.1002/14651858.CD007286.PUB5.
62. Eseonu CI, Eguia F, Garcia O, Kaplan PW, Quiñones-Hinojosa A. Comparative analysis of monotherapy versus duotherapy antiseizure drug management for postoperative seizure control in patients undergoing an awake craniotomy. J Neurosurg. 2018;128:1661–7.
63. Pourzitaki C, Tsaousi G, Apostolidou E, Karakoulas K, Kouvelas D, Amaniti E. Efficacy and safety of prophylactic levetiracetam in supratentorial brain tumour surgery: a systematic review and meta-analysis. Br J Clin Pharmacol. 2016;82(1):315–25.
64. Klimek M, van der Horst PH, Hoeks SE, Stolker RJ. Quality and quantity of memories in patients who undergo awake brain tumor resection. World Neurosurg. 2018;109:e258–64.
65. Elayat A, Jena SS, Nayak S, Sahu RN, Tripathy S. Enhanced recovery after surgery—ERAS in elective craniotomies-a non-randomized controlled trial. BMC Neurol. 2021;21:127. https://doi.org/10.1186/S12883-021-02150-7.
66. Wang Y, Xue YF, Zhao BF, Guo SC, Ji PG, Liu JH, Wang N, Chen F, Zhai YL, Wang Y, Xue YR. Real-world implementation of neurosurgical enhanced recovery after surgery (ERAS) protocol for glioma patients undergoing elective craniotomy. Front Oncol. 2022;12:860257.
67. Sanghvi D. Post-treatment imaging of high-grade gliomas. Indian J Radiol Imaging. 2015;25(02):102–8.
68. Gehring K, Sitskoorn MM, Gundy CM, Sikkes SA, Klein M, Postma TJ, Van Den Bent MJ, Beute GN, Enting RH, Kappelle AC, Boogerd W. Cognitive rehabilitation in patients with gliomas: a randomized, controlled trial. J Clin Oncol. 2009;27(22):3712–22.

The Role of Intraoperative Neurophysiologic Monitoring (IONM) in Awake Craniotomy<Intraoperative, Neuromonitoring, Awake Craniotomy>

Melisa Esmaeili and Hamidreza Rokhsatyazdy

1 Introduction

The eloquent area of the brain is responsible for verbal and written communication. Functional neuroimaging demonstrates inter-individual variability with the anatomical location of the brain's eloquent region. Some patients have shown functional contributions from areas located near, but outside the known traditional eloquent area. Traditionally, these areas adjacent to or close to the eloquent areas were thought to have little effect on written or spoken language skills; therefore, many neurosurgeons underestimated the impact of surgery on these regions. Now, it is understood that each patient has a unique known eloquent zone. This requires intraoperative cortical mapping to identify functions more accurately before removing brain tissue in patients undergoing epilepsy or brain tumor surgery in areas close to this region of the brain. The goal of intraoperative cortical mapping is to maximize surgical resection of the eloquent area while minimizing the incidence of permanent disability.

2 Intraoperative Neuromonitoring

Today, various methods of intraoperative neurophysiological monitoring are available to assess functions of the brain, brainstem, spinal cord, cranial nerves, and peripheral nerves during surgery. They play a valuable role in the diagnosis and prevention of nerve damage. Intraoperative monitoring has become a standard in neurosurgery today. Intraoperative neurophysiologic monitoring (IONM) records and monitors a wide range of physiological changes during the procedure [1, 2].

3 Awake Craniotomy

Awake craniotomy (AC) has been used to treat epilepsy for over a century. Currently, it is recognized as a standard procedure for various other surgeries, most prominently gliomas located within or close to the eloquent areas (i.e., sensorimotor or language

M. Esmaeili (✉)
Institute for Cognitive Science Studies, Tehran, Iran

H. Rokhsatyazdy
Department of Neurology, Shahid Beheshti University of Medical Science, Tehran, Iran

A. Pour-Rashidi, J. Aarabi (eds.), *The Principles of Successful Awake Craniotomy*,
https://doi.org/10.1007/978-981-99-2985-6_9

areas) of the brain [3]. Modern AC techniques employ IONM to identify and evaluate brain areas [4]. One of the primary goals of AC is maximal safe tumor resection without damaging healthy brain tissue. Cortical mapping is an important and useful technique to use during this process [5].

4 Motor Mapping and Monitoring Via Electrical Stimulation

For resection of lesions adjacent to Brodmann area 4, motor mapping can be used by direct electrical stimulation and identification of central sulcus (CS) via phase reversal technique (PRT). We use the latter as the starting point of motor mapping. After CS is identified, via somatosensory-evoked potential (SSEP) PRT, we proceed with direct electrical stimulation [6].

Direct electrical stimulation of primary motor cortex (PMC) at its depolarization threshold will produce compound muscle motor-evoked potentials (MEPs), also referred to in this chapter as muscle motor potentials evoked by direct cortical stimulation (DCS-MEPs). These will trigger selectively, depending upon the specific area on the motor homunculus where the current is applied. Stimulation at higher currents results in clinical movements [7].

Corticospinal tract (CST) can also be mapped via direct subcortical stimulation that will trigger the same MEPs. After mapping the eloquent cortical and subcortical structures, constant monitoring of these pathways can be achieved by continuous electrical stimulation of PMC. Changes from DCS-MEP prerejection baselines will be further interpreted. Alternatively, D waves can also be recorded at different spinal levels, via epidural electrodes. D waves represent the electrical volleys that are generated by direct stimulation of the PMC as they travel down the CST fibers. D waves are regarded as the most specific and reliable way to map and monitor the PMC [8–10].

4.1 Technical Method

4.1.1 Stimulation Technique

Three main methods of stimulation have been used for neurophysiologic cortical motor mapping: (a) the Penfield method was used earlier and included the Penfield paradigm with bipolar stimulation; (b) the most commonly used for motor mapping is the multi-pulse train technique via monopolar stimulation, also known as high-frequency anodal (cortical) or cathodal (subcortical) stimulation [11–13].

4.1.2 Penfield Method

The traditional technique, as described by Foster and Penfield as early as the 1930s, consists of repetitive pulses at 60 Hz, and 1 ms pulse width applied via a bipolar stimulation (handheld stimulator or two adjacent contacts of a subdural grid). However, slightly modified paradigms have also been used in clinical practice (e.g., 50 Hz) (Fig. 1 and 2) [11–13].

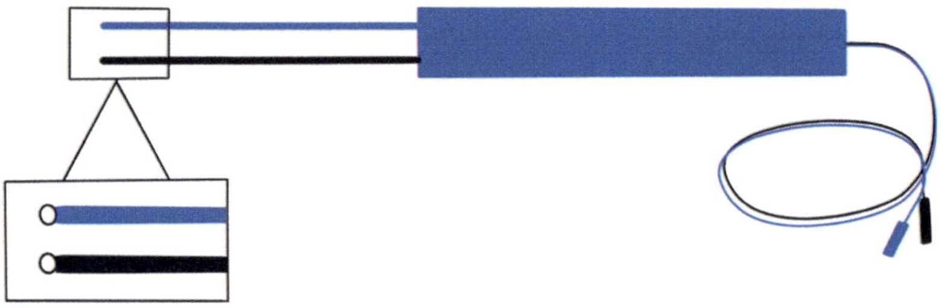

Fig. 1 Handheld ball tip bipolar stimulation probe used for motor mapping in the Penfield method (Jahangiri et al. This is an open-access article distributed under the terms of the Creative Commons Attribution License CC-BY 4.0., which permits unrestricted use, distribution, and reproduction in any medium, provided the original author and source are credited.) [12]

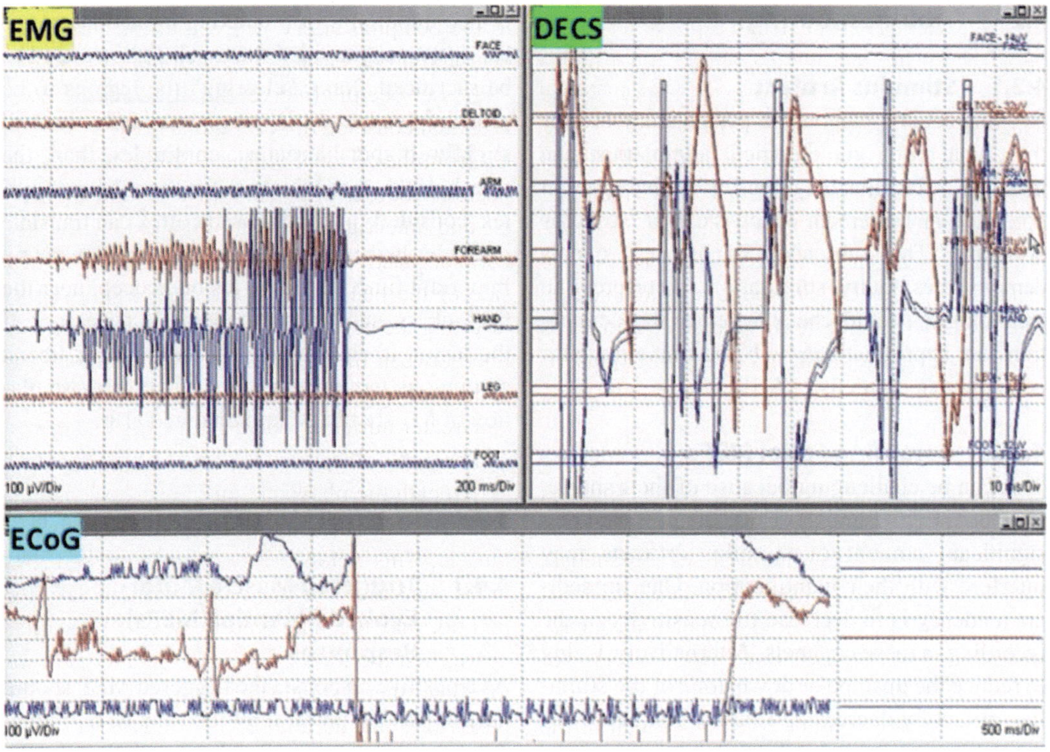

Fig. 2 Penfield motor mapping method. 50 Hz Penfield motor mapping evoked responses after bipolar manual stimulation. Several responses are recorded in the forearm and hand muscles. (Face: orbicularis oris; deltoid, arm: biceps brachii; Forearm: brachioradialis/flexor carpi ulnaris; Hand: abductor pollicis brevis/ abductor digit minimi; Leg: tibialis anterior; Foot: Illusion Abductor /EMG: electromyography; DECS: Penfield direct electrical stimulation of the cerebral cortex. ECoG: Electrocorticography) (Jahangiri et al. This is an open-access article distributed under the terms of the Creative Commons Attribution License CC-BY 4.0., which permits unrestricted use, distribution, and reproduction in any medium, provided the original author and source are credited.) [12]

4.1.3 Multipoles Train Method

The high-frequency anodal stimulation paradigm, also known as the multipoles train technique, efficiently depolarizes M1, triggering MEPs. It consists of applying a train or trains (e.g., 1 Hz) of brief pulses (i.e., 0.5 ms pulse width), each train consisting of 4–6 pulses at high frequency (250–500 Hz) with intensities ranging from 1 to 25 mA. We use constant current stimulation; however, constant voltage stimulation can also be used. Both monopolar and bipolar stimulation can be applied. High-frequency anodal stimulation is superior to other methods in cortical motor mapping, and it monitors three key elements: monopolar, anodal active stimulation, and high-frequency p pulses [13].

High-frequency stimulation introduced an additional net advantage in motor mapping under general anesthesia by allowing rapid and effective summation of the excitatory postsynaptic potentials at the level of the alpha motor neuron and thus, the efficient depolarization of the latter [14].

Ultimately, monopolar stimulation is superior to bipolar stimulation, allowing motor mapping at lower thresholds [15]. Higher specificity of the location of the MEPs and reduction of noise during recording is achieved by placing two needle electrodes per muscle (rather than one needle per muscle) and displaying one muscle activity per channel. Most importantly, having two needles per muscle will increase our sensitivity in identifying a triggered electrophysiologic response in that muscle [16].

4.2 Troubleshooting

4.2.1 Stimulus Artifact

Evoking action potentials in peripheral nerves or the spinal cord via electrical stimulation can make an artifact that may interfere with the action potentials measurement which is called "stimulus artifact". The absence of these signals demonstrates faulty stimulation; therefore, the technologist should check whether the connections are appropriate and whether the stimulator is plugged in correctly [17–19].

4.2.2 Recording Facial MEPs

This can be challenging because of their shorter latencies (Figs. 1 and 2). Thus, the presence of a significant amount of stimulus artifacts may interfere with their identification. One immediate tendency is to decrease the sensitivity of the recording in these channels. Alternatively, trying to reduce the upslope or downslope of the stimulus artifact by decreasing the low-frequency filter (LFF) can be helpful. A third option is to change the stimulus parameters so that the "length" of the stimulus artifact is shortened, and the latter does not superimpose on the responses of the MEPs [17–19].

4.2.3 Noisy Muscle Channels

This could impair the identification of the lower amplitude MEPs. As a consequence, to be able to distinguish evoked motor potentials, one should stimulate at a high stimulus amplitude, probably higher than the actual primary motor mapping threshold. To eliminate 60 Hz, such as changing the existing ground electrode or adding one on that limb [17–19].

4.3 Procedure and Interpretation of Results

Our initial approach is by identifying the PMC or M1 at its threshold (positive mapping). Identification of the supplementary motor regions is also important for predicting immediate surgical outcome, provided that such regions need to be sacrificed. Next, "clearing" the regions to be resected (negative mapping) is usually done at slightly higher stimulus amplitudes than the threshold (1–2 mA higher) for the eloquent cortex, considering that diseased cortex can translate into elevated stimulation threshold yet retain important function. If the lesion is deep, near the CST fibers, subcortical mapping is necessary. If the lesion is either near M1 and/or CST fibers, continuous motor monitoring via direct stimulation of M1 should be implemented [18].

4.4 Cortical Motor Mapping

4.4.1 Triggered Muscle Motor-Evoked Potential (MEPs) Responses

As a positive response, the triggered MEP should have at least 50 μV in amplitude and be reproducible in subsequent stimulations [19–20]. We believe that polyphasic morphology is a sign of reliable activation of the motor pathways. However, consistent, high-amplitude, normal latency biphasic/triphasic responses are also seen. The reliability of the mapping results is further confirmed by remaining "blinded" to the cortical location of each stimulation. Normal variations of the latencies, amplitudes, and widths of the mMEPs are seen within different regions of the motor cortex.

4.4.2 Importance of Motor Mapping at M1 Threshold

If the stimulation is done with too high stimulus amplitudes, the motor response triggered may be due to the spreading of the current to the cortex adjacent to the stimulated region. Highly specific localization of certain parts of the motor strip may be particularly important for the placement of cortical epidural stimulators for the treatment of intractable pain localized in a very specific area [19–20].

5 Primary Somatosensory Function Mapping and Monitoring

This section addresses specifically the mapping and monitoring of the primary somatosensory regions. Mapping of the primary somatosensory areas in the postcentral regions can be done with the patient awake or under anesthesia [17].

5.1 Technical Methods

5.1.1 Stimulation Technique

To trigger sensory symptoms, electrical cortical stimulation can be done with either multipole training or Penfield methods.

5.1.2 Recording Responses

While the patient is awake sensory symptoms are the endpoint of stimulation. However, as in the case of the CS localization, mapping of the somatosensory cortex could also be done by recording the thalamocortical, usually median SSEPs over the ipsilateral hemisphere while stimulating the contralateral (e.g., median) nerve at the wrist.

5.1.3 Electrocorticography (ECOG) Recordings

ECOG recordings are essential if cortical electrical stimulation is applied (to trigger sensory symptoms) [21].

6 Central Sulcus Localization

Sensorimotor mapping starts with accurate identification of the CS. The CS can be identified on the 1.5 T MRI images by using anatomic landmarks such as the intersection between the superior frontal sulcus with the pre-CS (sagittal images); the motor hand area as the omega-shaped knob (axial images) or hook-like configuration (sagittal images). However, one of the most reliable tools for identifying CS is the use of MSSEP PRT. Overall, this technique is based on the sudden reversal in polarity of the median thalamocortical SSEPs, at the level of the CS. At approximately 19–20 ms after the stimulation of the contralateral (to the hemisphere operated on) median nerve at the wrist, the postcentral primary somatosensory parietal cortex becomes more electronegative than the precentral frontal region, creating a dipole-oriented perpendicular to the CS, from posterior toward anterior regions [22–24].

6.1 Technical Methods

6.1.1 Stimulation Technique

The contralateral median nerve at the wrist is the most commonly used stimulation site for this method. Because the SSEP phase reversal could be seen along the extent of the CS, other peripheral nerves can also be stimulated. For example, when lesions are present along the motor cortex near the interhemispheric fissure, the femoral nerve can also be stimulated for motor strip mapping. For this method of treatment, needle electrodes can be inserted over the contralateral inguinal ligament, approximately 15 mm lateral to the femoral artery. The femoral nerve is stimulated with increasing intensities until small twitches are noted in the quadriceps femoris. Nevertheless, the most common nerve in the lower extremity used for stimulation and SSEP recording is the posterior tibial nerve, the peroneal, and ulnar nerves.

Median SSEPs have a robust morphology and good amplitudes, and thus are relatively easy to obtain. For stimulation, two disposable conductive solid-gel electrodes, with attached 1.5 mm safety lead wires (Rochester, Electro-Medical Inc.), are attached to the skin overlying the contralateral (to the hemisphere of interest) median nerve at the wrist, along its length. The electrical stimulus delivered is a rectangular pulse of 0.3 ms width, delivered at a frequency of 3.17 Hz, with a progressive increase in the intensity until thumb muscle twitches are observed (needed amplitude varies between 10 and 25 mA) [22–24].

6.1.2 Recording Technique

We have found it very useful to first record a baseline scalp median SSEPs at the beginning of the case. This is done from the usual centroparietal locations. For direct cortical SSEP recordings, we use a platinum strip electrode (Ad-Tech subdural strip electrodes), placed by the surgeon directly on the contralateral cortex (can also be placed epidurally), in a direction perpendicular to it. The contact diameter is 2.3 mm, the intercontact distance is 10 mm, and the total length of the strip is about 90 mm. The stimulated peripheral nerve should indicate the location of this strip on the convexity. When the femoral or posterior tibial nerves are stimulated, the recording strip should be along the superior lip of the interhemispheric fissure. Our reference electrode is either a subdermal needle (anesthetized patients) or a surface stick-on (awake patients) electrode, placed on the contralateral mastoid.

If MSSEP PRT is attempted during phase II invasive recordings for epilepsy surgery evaluation, it has been our experience that identifying the row of electrodes that is appropriate or sufficiently well positioned relative to the presumed location of the CS is very often unsuccessful given the random orientation of the implanted subdural grid in that respect. The usual recording parameters employed are the following: time base 5–7 ms/div; sensitivity 10 μV/div. By default, our method includes both references (each strip electrode referenced to the ipsilateral montages) [22–24].

6.1.3 Troubleshooting

- *60 Hz noise and other types.* One of the most common problems with this technique is the significant amount of 60 Hz artifact introduced into the recording. Even when such direct cortical recordings are expected to yield high-amplitude-evoked potentials, the signal-to-noise ratio can be significantly degraded in the presence of 60 Hz noise.

Turning on the 60 Hz filter notch can help. It should be ensured that the signal obtained is of maximum amplitude, and that the stimulation is adequate: a good twitch of the thumb is a sure sign of adequate stimulation. The stimulus frequency must be a number that does not exactly divide the 60 Hz (for example, we use 3.17 Hz, not 3 Hz). Unstable contacts can lead to increased rejection or decreased signal-to-noise ratio by introducing significant amounts of noise. Therefore, an impedance check should be performed. Irrigation of the contacts with saline usually improves any impedance.

7 Intraoperative Neurophysiologic Monitoring and Mapping of the Visual Pathways

Visual pathways are critical structures carrying visual information from the eye (retina) to the occipital lobes. Thus, orbital, trans-sphenoidal, parasellar, cortical (parietal, temporal, and occipital), and endoscopic procedures can result in their manipulation and damage. Preserving eyesight is of key interest during such surgeries [25–26].

Intraoperative monitoring of the visual pathways via visual-evoked potentials (VEPs) would help avert postoperative complications such as diminished to total loss of visual function. Obtaining reliable and reproducible intraoperative VEPs used for continuous monitoring of visual pathways under general anesthesia has been challenging. Mapping the visual pathway is increasingly challenging with little information. Other researchers were able to electrically stimulate the optic tract or optic radiations triggering both positive and negative visual symptoms as well as VEPs recorded via scalp electrodes (Fig. 3) [25–27].

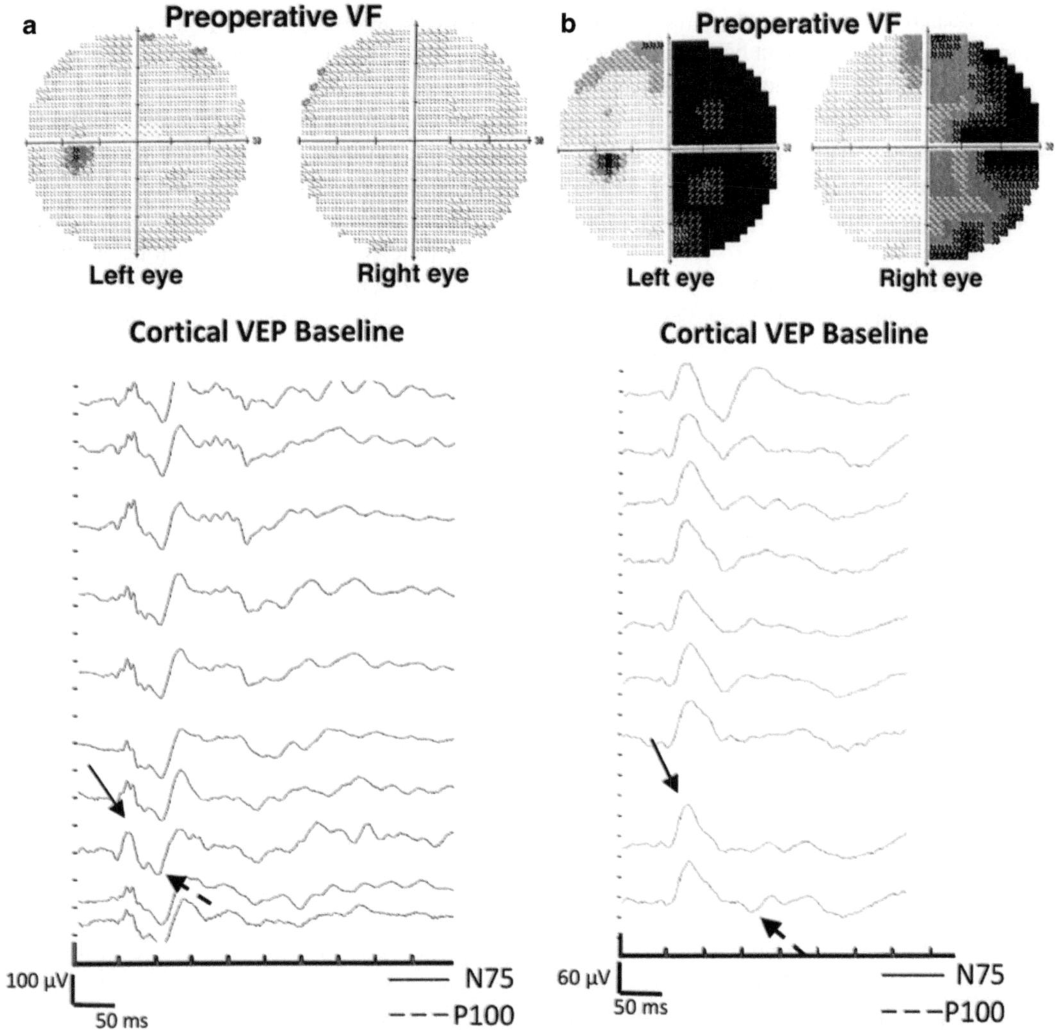

Fig. 3 Basal cortical VEP recordings were performed using subdural electrodes at the occipital pole in a patient with intact preoperative visual field (VF) (**a**) and in a patient with significant VF deficit (**b**). Note the similar VEP appearance regardless of VF status (License Number: 5470091224860) [25]

7.1 Stimulation Technique

7.1.1 Pattern Shift Stimulation

This is the most sensitive technique for the detection of conduction defects. It also has less intra- and interindividual variability of the recorded VEPs, both for amplitudes as well as latencies. The visual stimulus is presented as a checkerboard on a computer screen with constant luminescence. The black and white check dimensions can be modified depending upon a patient's visual acuity (VA) as it can be their alternating frequency. The smaller the checks the higher their sensitivity to detect VEP abnormalities. Nevertheless, the smaller the checks the more affected the recordings by decreased VA. For example, a standard check size is 15 inches, corresponding to a 3 mm side check presented on a board situated 70 cm in front of the patient. A patient with VA of 20/20 can be presented with a checkerboard with a 5 inches check size of 4 mm presented at 275 cm in front of him or her; whereas a patient with a VA of 20/100 can be tested with a 30′ check size presented 50 cm in front of him or her [25].

7.1.2 Flash Stimulation

Flash stimulation is known to be less sensitive for detecting conduction defects in the visual pathways with direct clinical implications. This explains the relatively high number of reported false negative cases. Although no clear flash VEP (fVEP) changes were reported intraoperatively, the patients did awaken from surgery with new visual deficits. In this manner, high-intensity flashes may provide responses that are better indicators of the visual function than the lower intensity. Another reason for the high number of false negatives is the inability to perform preferential hemifield stimulations, thus detecting a postchiasmatic lesion of the ipsilateral optic tract or parts of the optic radiation [26].

Despite the aforementioned shortcomings, fVEPs remain the only ones that do not require the patient's cooperation and thus can be used under general anesthesia. An ideal stimulating device would be a soft round silicone disc with LED lights embedded. Typically, the stimulating device is taped over the closed eyelid. This would ensure that the device sits well over the closed eyelid. Another factor that could result in fVEPs fluctuations is the variation of the retinal reaction to light, with greater responses in the initial period of flashlight stimulation. Thus, to obtain a steady retinal activation, an initial period of 1-min stimulation is recommended before fVEP monitoring is initiated. Using electroretinogram or electroretinography (ERG) to ensure that the light falls properly on it and thus adequately stimulates the retina [26].

7.2 Recording Technique

- *Electroretinography.* Subdermal needle electrodes can be used for recording the ERG, with the active electrode placed at the lateral canthus and the reference electrode placed at Fz.
- *B1. Flash Visual Evoked Potentials.* Typically scalp electrodes are used for recording the intraoperative VEPs. Following the 10–20 system the recording electrodes are placed at the following locations: mastoids (i.e., A1, A2), Fz, Cz, Pz, Oz, O1, O2, L10, and R10. O1 and O2 (also known as L5 and R5) are placed at 5 cm from Oz, on the left and right occipital areas respectively. L10 and R10 are placed at 10 cm to the left and right of Oz. The most commonly used recording channels are Oz–Fz, O1–Fz, O2–Fz, L10–Fz, R10–Fz, and Pz–Fz. In general, the maximum P100 amplitudes are in Oz–Fz or Oz– Cz channels. This is because the area of maximal negativity can be anywhere between Fz and Cz. However, Pz can also become electronegative so that the phase reversal will occur between Cz and Pz. Of note, in VEP recordings, both Fz and the mastoids are active references, given their electronegative charge. Fz is placed approximately 12 cm above nasion and will show a negative peak at approximately 100 ms. fVEP recordings have also been performed directly from the optic nerve.
- *B2. Recording Parameters.* The recordings are done at a LFF range of 1–30 Hz, with a high-frequency filter (HFF) range of 100–300 Hz. An LFF of 10–30 Hz will also shorten the amplifier recovery time after the effect of electrocautery.

7.3 Anesthesia Method

In these surgeries, anesthesia should use several methods to keep the patient awake during the surgery. One of the most important points during anesthesia is the quick return of the patient's consciousness, full awareness, and full cooperation with the surgical team to perform the surgery, which plays a very important role in the success rate of the operation [28].

To induce anesthesia, specialists usually use propofol as a target-controlled infusion (TCI) along with a narcotic [29]. At this stage, the experience of the anesthesiologist is very important because the reaction of each patient to the drugs received is different, and therefore, must be able to establish a balance between the anesthetic agents to achieve the best result because any disruption could interfere with the patient's performance and cooperation. Postoperatively, the results can be very effective. Equally important to consider is that the anesthetic used will affect the mapping process [30].

In AC, during general anesthesia neither a tracheal tube nor mechanical ventilation are used; however, moderated anesthesia (use of laryngeal mask airway, LMA) is used, which reduces the number of complications and hemodynamic changes in the patient. There are two common methods for performing anesthesia in AC such as monitored anesthesia care (MAC) and asleep-awake-asleep (AAA). Among the most common complications after surgery in these patients, are seizures, increased blood pressure, respiratory depression, nausea and vomiting, and cerebral edema [30].

8 Conclusion

Intraoperative neurophysiologic motor mapping and monitoring are essential for achieving safe maximal resection of lesions near eloquent cortical and subcortical regions. A multimodality approach, neurophysiology expertise, preoperative planning, and multidisciplinary collaboration will all significantly increase its reliability and safety.

References

1. Hande VH, Gunasekaran H, Hegde S, Shashidhar A, Arimappamagan A. Role of clinical neuropsychologists in awake-craniotomy. Neurol India. 2021;69(3):711.
2. Yamao Y, Matsumoto R, Kikuchi T, Yoshida K, Kunieda T, Miyamoto S. Intraoperative brain mapping by cortico-cortical evoked potential. Front Hum Neurosci. 2021;15:635453.
3. Lemée JM, Bernard F, Ter Minassian A, Menei P. Right hemisphere cognitive functions: from clinical and anatomical bases to brain mapping during awake craniotomy. Part II: neuropsychological tasks and brain mapping. World Neurosurg. 2018;118:360–7.
4. Bernard F, Lemée JM, Ter Minassian A, Menei P. Right hemisphere cognitive functions: from clinical and anatomic bases to brain mapping during awake craniotomy part I: clinical and functional anatomy. World Neurosurg. 2018;118:348–59.
5. Zhang JJ, Lee KS, Voisin MR, Hervey-Jumper SL, Berger MS, Zadeh G. Awake craniotomy for resection of supratentorial glioblastoma: a systematic review and meta-analysis. Neuro-Oncol Adv. 2020;2(1):vdaa111.
6. Minahan RE. Intraoperative neuromonitoring. Neurologist. 2002;8(4):209–26.
7. Yang S, Zhou L, Lu Z, Ma B, Ji Q, Wang Y. Systematic review with meta-analysis of intraoperative neuromonitoring during thyroidectomy. Int J Surg. 2017;39:104–13.
8. Oh T, Nagasawa DT, Fong BM, Trang A, Gopen Q, Parsa AT, Yang I. Intraoperative neuromonitoring techniques in the surgical management of acoustic neuromas. Neurosurg Focus. 2012;33(3):E6.
9. Rahimpour S, Friedman AH, Fukushima T, Zomorodi AR. Microsurgical resection of vestibular schwannomas: complication avoidance. J Neuro-Oncol. 2016;130(2):367–75.
10. Liu SW, Jiang W, Zhang HQ, Li XP, Wan XY, Emmanuel B, Shu K, Chen JC, Chen J, Lei T. Intraoperative neuromonitoring for removal of large vestibular schwannoma: facial nerve outcome and predictive factors. Clin Neurol Neurosurg. 2015;133:83–9.
11. Calancie B. Intraoperative neuromonitoring and alarm criteria for judging MEP responses to transcranial electric stimulation: the threshold-level method. J Clin Neurophysiol. 2017;34(1):12–21.
12. Jahangiri FR, Liang M, Kabir SS, et al. Motor mapping of the brain: Taniguchi versus Penfield method. Cureus. 2022;14(5):e24901. https://doi.org/10.7759/cureus.24901.
13. Chacko S, McCann ME, Soriano SG. Surgery for scoliosis. In: Koht, Sloan, Toleikis's monitoring the nervous system for anesthesiologists and other health care professionals. Cham: Springer; 2023. p. 591–601.
14. Shils JL, Sloan TB. Intraoperative neuromonitoring. Int Anesthesiol Clin. 2015;53(1):53–73.
15. Sloan T. Anesthesia and intraoperative neurophysiological monitoring in children. Childs Nerv Syst. 2010;26(2):227–35.
16. You H, Qiao H. Intraoperative neuromonitoring during resection of gliomas involving eloquent areas. Front Neurol. 2021;12:952.
17. Giussani C, Roux FE, Ojemann J, Sganzerla EP, Pirillo D, Papagno C. Is preoperative functional magnetic resonance imaging reliable for language areas mapping in brain tumor surgery? Review of language functional magnetic resonance imaging and direct

cortical stimulation correlation studies. Neurosurgery. 2010;66(1):113–20.
18. Zhou Q, Li M, Yi L, He B, Li X, Jiang Y. Intraoperative neuromonitoring during brain arteriovenous malformation microsurgeries and postoperative dysfunction: a retrospective follow-up study. Medicine. 2017;96(39):e8054.
19. Southwell DG, Hervey-Jumper SL, Perry DW, Berger MS. Intraoperative mapping during repeat awake craniotomy reveals the functional plasticity of adult cortex. J Neurosurg. 2016;124(5):1460–9.
20. Duffau H. Stimulation mapping of white matter tracts to study brain functional connectivity. Nat Rev Neurol. 2015;11(5):255–65.
21. Morsy AA. Resective epilepsy surgery with intraoperative brain mapping techniques: experiences from a multidisciplinary epilepsy team in Egypt East Afr J Neurol Sci 2022;1(Supp 1).
22. Rofes A, Miceli G. Language mapping with verbs and sentences in awake surgery: a review. Neuropsychol Rev. 2014;24(2):185–99.
23. Duffau H. Awake surgery for nonlanguage mapping. Neurosurgery. 2010;66(3):523–9.
24. Noll K, Asman P, Connelly K, Tasnim I, Swamy C, Ene C, Sudhakar T, Grasu R, Liu HL, Kumar V, Muir M. NCOG-14 Intraoperative cognitive-linguistic mapping guided by visualization of gamma band modulation electrocorticograms: proof of concept in a patient with left temporal and occipital low-grade astrocytoma. Neuro-Oncology. 2022;24(Supplement_7):Vii200.
25. de Melo MN, Verst SM. Evoked potential–visual pathways approach beyond visual evoked potentials. In: Intraoperative monitoring. Cham: Springer; 2022. p. 143–63.
26. Rajashekar D, Lavrador JP, Ghimire P, Keeble H, Harris L, Pereira N, Patel S, Beyh A, Gullan R, Ashkan K, Bhangoo R. Simultaneous motor and visual intraoperative neuromonitoring in asleep parietal lobe surgery: dual strip technique. J Pers Med. 2022;12(9):1478.
27. Lavrador JP, Gioti I, Hoppe S, Jung J, Patel S, Gullan R, Ashkan K, Bhangoo R, Vergani F. Altered motor excitability in patients with diffuse gliomas involving motor eloquent areas: the impact of tumor grading. Neurosurgery. 2021;88(1):183–92.
28. Huncke K, Van de Wiele B, Fried I, Rubinstein EH. The asleep-awake-asleep anesthetic technique for intraoperative language mapping. Neurosurgery. 1998;42(6):1312–6.
29. Liou JY, Wang HY, Tsou MY, Chang WK, Kuo IT, Ting CK. Opioid and propofol pharmacodynamics modeling during brain mapping in awake craniotomy. J Chin Med Assoc. 2019;82(5):390–5.
30. Kulikov A, Lubnin A. Anesthesia for awake craniotomy. Curr Opin Anesthesiol. 2018;31(5):506–10.

Neurocognition in Awake Craniotomy<Cognition, Neural Network, Awake Craniotomy>

Sajad Haghshenas and Fatemeh Sadat Mirfazeli

1 Principles in Neurocognition

1.1 Cognitive Function

Neurocognitive functions (NCF) are brain-based skills that are connected to specific areas in the brain and are needed in the acquisition of knowledge, manipulation of information, reasoning, and processing of thoughts. Cognitive neuropsychologists broadly study NCF to understand how the structure and function of the brain relate to cognition and behavior in normal and pathological cases [1]. Some of these neurocognitive domains include language, spatial awareness, learning, sensory perception, comprehension, memory, executive function, working memory, and motor skills. Such functions are generally specialized, but they also overlap or interact with each other, and there is a degree of modularity in brain cognitive functions.

1.2 Cognitive Impairment

Cognitive impairment is an inclusive term that refers to the reduction of cognitive function when physical changes have occurred in the brain. Cognitive impairment in the brain is either the result of aging or a neurological or mental illness [2, 3]. Assessing cognitive impairment is a method to measure the severity and burden of epilepsy, brain tumors, Parkinson's disease, and other neurological disorders [2, 3].

Clinical neuropsychologists may specialize in neuroscience assessments to detect and understand such deficits and they are involved in the rehabilitation of an affected person [3]. Cognitive symptoms are common in patients with brain tumors [4, 5]. Timely identification of problems with NCF is an important aspect of medical care, as cognition is critical for complex activities of daily living, work, and functional independence, thus playing a critical role in the quality of life [5]. In patients with tumors or neurological problems who need surgery, neuropsychological assessment is necessary to accurately understand the impact of brain disorders [4, 5].

2 Neural Network in the Brain

Large-scale neural networks are thought to be an essential substrate for the implementation of cognitive function by the brain [6]. This idea has emerged from a thorough understanding of cognition along with the knowledge of how large-scale neurocognitive networks operate [6]. Such understanding requires insight into structural,

S. Haghshenas (✉)
Shahid Beheshti University of Medical Sciences, Institute of Cognitive Science Studies, Tehran, Iran

F. S. Mirfazeli
Iran University of Medical Sciences, Tehran, Iran
e-mail: mirfazeli.f@iums.ac.ir

A. Pour-Rashidi, J. Aarabi (eds.), *The Principles of Successful Awake Craniotomy*,
https://doi.org/10.1007/978-981-99-2985-6_10

functional, and dynamical aspects of network operations, and the intimate interweaving of which may be responsible for the intricacies of cognition [6].

Knowledge of anatomical structure is basic to understanding how neurocognitive networks operate. Phylogenetically and ontogenetically determined patterns of synaptic connectivity form a structural network of brain areas, allowing communication between widely distributed collections of areas [6]. The function of neurocognitive networks depends on selective activation of anatomically linked cortical and subcortical areas in a wide variety of configurations. Large-scale functional networks provide cooperative processing which gives expression to cognitive function. The dynamics of neurocognitive network function relate to the evolving patterns of interacting brain areas that express cognitive function in real-time [6, 7]. Basic similarity of the structural, functional, and dynamical features of all neurocognitive networks in the brain causes them to function according to common operational principles [7].

The formation of neural context through the coordinated mutual constraint of multiple interacting cortical areas is considered as a guiding principle underlying all cognitive functions. Increasing knowledge of the operating principles of neurocognitive networks is likely to promote the advancement of cognitive theories and to seed strategies for the enhancement of cognitive abilities [6].

The gap between knowledge of the brain and mind can be narrowed by understanding the neural systems that perform cognitive operations. According to this perspective, the neurocognitive network is a critical concept for combining neuroscience and cognitive science [6]. Neurocognitive networks are integrated large-scale neural systems that execute high-level brain functions of which cognition is comprised. Although a multitude of varieties exist in their expression, it is not unreasonable that these networks should follow common laws of operation, given the neuroanatomical and neurophysiological similarity that is present throughout the brain [6].

The anatomical architecture of the network provides the basic substrate of interconnected brain regions that, by way of their interactions, can express functions that are different depending on the specific subsets of connected regions that cooperate. The functions of the neurocognitive network are expressed in real-time by the coordinated actions of cooperating areas, with the states of coordination changing dynamically [6, 7]. In this process, the active states of neurocognitive networks are selectively structured in three key dimensions. First, they are spatially structured by the combined activation of discrete, local cortical, and subcortical neuronal assemblies. Next, they are temporally structured by the changing combinatorial arrangement of active assemblies during the expression of cognitive functions. Finally, they are coordinatively structured by specifically patterned joint actions of activated assemblies. The presumption that neurocognitive networks do in fact implement cognitive function further implies that the expression of cognitive function occurs as structured states, with a structure corresponding to that of the active states of neurocognitive networks. Thus, by careful examination of the anatomical, functional, and dynamical aspects of neurocognitive networks, we anticipate the eventual emergence of a neural language for describing cognition [6].

2.1 Anatomical Structure of the Neurocognitive Networks

We consider the anatomical organization of neurocognitive networks to be of prime importance in shaping the cognitive operations of the brain. Neural networks may be described on various scales, from small assemblies of neurons to the whole brain [6].

2.2 Functional Expression of Neurocognitive Networks

The intricate anatomical connectivity of the cerebral cortex provides the basis for an enormous space of possible combinations of co-active areas. The guiding concept in this section is that the functional expression of a cognitive operation requires co-activation of a specific combination of interconnected local area networks. The co-activated local area networks represent a subset of the total set of possible networks in the cerebral cortex [6].

2.3 Dynamics of Neurocognitive Networks

Neurocognitive networks are flexibly adaptive to the rapidly changing computational demands of cognitive processing (Bressler 1995). This adaptivity requires that the neurocognitive network be able to organize and reorganize in different patterns of coordination as computationally required on a sub-second time scale [6].

Assessment of cognitive features requires retrospectively assessing neurological deficits, subjective concerns from patient or caregiver, and cognitive deficits at baseline and post-surgery for patients with newly diagnosed low-grade glioma (LGG) who underwent baseline neuropsychological evaluation and magnetic resonance imaging before awake craniotomy (AC) [8].

2.4 Impairment of Neurocognitive Function in Patients with Brain Tumors

Deficits in NCF occur in 90% of patients with supratentorial brain tumors at varying points in the disease course [9, 10]. At the time of diagnosis, these deficits may be related to the tumor disrupting both local and distant brain networks [9]. Mechanisms of these effects include direct tissue damage via necrosis, compression of neural structures due to mass effect from tumor and surrounding edema, and infiltrative growth into critical fiber pathways and networks [5]. Neurosurgical intervention can alleviate some of these symptoms, particularly when resection reduces mass effect but can also cause additional NCF symptoms if critical brain regions or pathways are damaged during surgery. Strategies to reduce the risk of neurosurgical deficits, such as functional MRI and awake craniotomies with intraoperative mapping, have improved these outcomes.

Chemotherapy is also known to contribute to cognitive decline in patients with both primary brain tumors (e.g., about 30% of patients have been shown to have NCF changes after chemotherapy treatment in the absence of disease progression) and brain metastases. The complex interplay of these multiple etiologies of NCF dysfunction in patients with brain tumors implies that consistent cognitive assessment and monitoring throughout the course of disease is an important part of comprehensive clinical care. Diverse approaches to management may be necessary at different intervals in the disease course and typically require a multidisciplinary approach [5, 11].

3 Necessity for Neurocognitive Tests

The use of intraoperative monitoring and neuroscience tests of cognitive functions before, during, and after awake surgery is new, and this technique has undergone far-reaching changes in recent years, especially in the context of glioma surgery. In fact, this rapid development has brought about greater awareness from neurosurgeons and neuropsychiatrists that preserving the quality of life for patients with a long survival expectancy (as in LGGs) cannot be reduced only to the assessment of functions whose damage leads to overt consequences, such as aphasia or motor defects [12]. As a result, the intraoperative mapping, and neuropsychological tests of other important cognitive functions (e.g., socio-cognitive functions, spatial cognition, and semantic cognition) in both hemispheres have been advocated to provide patients the best opportunities of resuming a normal socio-professional life quickly after surgery. Concomitantly, as stimulation mapping using direct electrostimulation is the only available technique permitting both real-time anatomical functional correlations and interrogation of white matter fiber connectivity from a functional standpoint, considerable progress has been made in understanding the role of neural pathway in cognition and behavior. This has led to the development of neuropsychological-based and anatomically constrained models of several human functions in which neuroplasticity has been considered [12].

Prior to experience in intraoperative cognitive mapping and neuro-scientific tests, researchers have described different behavioral paradigms and tests typically used in awake surgery as well as how they are selected and modulated to identify and spare critical brain-wide cognitive systems of the brain. A discussion on how to improve intraoperative cognitive mapping and tests, while recognizing their merits and limitations, is provided. Knowledge gained in this chapter may also aid neuropsychologists and neurosurgeons to better cope with both the functional and anatomical connections of the brain, and their reorganization potential from a network perspective [12].

In AC, it is important to maximize the extent of resection of both low-LGGs and high-grade gliomas (HGG). Gross total resection (GTR) relates to longer progression-free survival and reduced incidence of relapse [11, 13]. It is necessary to save as much functional brain tissue as possible to achieve this optimal outcome without long-lasting deterioration of language, motor, or NCF while preserving the highest quality of life [11, 13].

The current gold standard during resections of LGGs located in language-eloquent areas is AC combined with neuro-scientific tests, intraoperative stimulation mapping (ISM), and cognitive neuromonitoring [13]. This technique can minimize permanent postoperative deficits while maximizing the extent of resection, especially in cases of infiltrative tumors such as LGG, in which the greater the resection, the longer the patient survival [13].

Few studies have examined the effects of AC in patients with HGGs. Evaluation of cognitive neuroscience and neuropsychological outcome has received insufficient emphasis in clinical practices. Language has been the domain most frequently examined. However, it is not clear if patients with HGG have the same trend of language recovery as patients with LGG. Moreover, to date, there are no established standards for evaluation of postoperative deficits in other cognitive domains. Results from different studies are too arbitrary and heterogeneous to draw definite conclusions about the cognitive course after surgery [13, 14].

4 Cognitive Assessment in Brain Tumors

In surgery for tumors of the brain, attention is devoted to the quality of resection and preservation of cognitive abilities and functions. Besides monitoring tumor variables (size, location, histology, edema), a multifaceted battery of tests has been used to investigate mood, cognition, and language to assess the burden of disease and treatment, as well as the relationships between these three dimensions [15]. A general decline in postoperative cognitive performance (significant for memory and attention only) and language function (significant for picture naming) was observed. Cognitive assessment performed in conjunction with language testing is a necessary step in the global evaluation of brain tumor patients both before and after surgery [15].

Cognitive symptoms occur in almost all patients with brain tumors at varying points of the disease [16, 17]. Deficits in NCF may be caused by the tumor itself, treatment (surgery, radiation, or chemotherapy), or other complicating factors (e.g., seizures, fatigue, mood disturbance) and can have a profound effect on functional independence and quality of life. Assessment of NCF is an important part of comprehensive care of patients with brain tumors. In the neurosurgery clinic, assessments may include cognitive screening tools and inquiry into subjective cognitive function. Neuropsychological and neuroscience assessment is an important adjunct to identify cognitive symptoms and can be used as an opportunity to intervene through transformative feedback and treatment planning. Preventative measures can be taken to reduce cognitive side effects of treatment, such as awake craniotomies with cognitive intraoperative mapping during neurosurgery or prophylactic measures during radiation therapy (e.g., hippocampal avoidance, and neuroprotectant treatment with memantine). Rehabilitative therapies, including cognitive rehabilitation and computerized cognitive exercise, are options for managing cognitive problems in an individualized manner. Identification and management of co-occurring issues, such as sleep disturbance, fatigue, and depression, can also improve NCF. There are promising therapies under development that may provide new options for treatment in the future. Integrating careful assessment and treatment of cognition throughout the disease course for patients with brain tumors can improve functional outcomes and quality of life [5].

5 Practical Applications

- Difficulties with NCF occur in up to 90% of patients with brain tumors at some point during the disease process and are a major detractor from the overall quality of life.
- Screening procedures in the neuro-surgery clinic may include brief objective measures, such as the Montreal Cognitive Assessment, but these have limited sensitivity and should be augmented by subjective cognitive assessment using surveys.
- Cognitive neuroscience and neuropsychological evaluations are sensitive and useful tools to identify NCF difficulties and provide opportunities to improve understanding of cognitive problems and develop individualized treatment plans.
- Cognitive rehabilitation conducted by a therapist is an effective method for NCF improvement using compensatory strategies and assistive devices. Computerized/automated cognitive "exercise" approaches have limited evidence of benefit at this time [5].

5.1 Assessment of Neurocognitive Symptoms

Monitoring for NCF deficits or changes is a challenge for neurosurgery clinicians, given the numerous neurologic and medical issues that must be managed in brief visits. This difficulty is complicated by the fact that brief NCF screening measures, such as the Mini-Mental State Examination (MMSE) and the Montreal Cognitive Assessment (MoCA) have limited sensitivity to subtle but meaningful changes in NCF that people with brain tumors experience [5]. Despite these limitations, neurosurgeons often must resort to these screening tools as the only feasible options for in-clinic performance-based assessment of NCF. To enhance sensitivity to subtle changes in cognition, clinicians often use brief self-report surveys to assess subjective NCF symptoms, along with other quality-of-life issues. Commonly used scales include the Functional Assessment for Cancer Therapy-Brain (FACT-Br) and the European Organization for Research and Treatment of Cancer (EORTC) Quality of Life Scale [5]. These measures can generate specific indices of NCF. If administered consistently over time, changes in function may be apparent to the clinician, which can prompt referral for more in-depth evaluations [5, 18–20].

The gold standard for NCF assessment is comprehensive cognitive neuroscience and neuropsychological evaluation [19]. Multidisciplinary brain tumor clinics are increasingly integrating cognitive neuropsychiatrists as members of the patient care team, providing access to detailed assessments. In the context of brain tumor management, neuroscience, and neuropsychological evaluations may be abbreviated from a traditional battery of tests and tailored to individual patient needs and levels of functioning. These assessments can identify NCF changes before visible changes on brain imaging and are prognostic of overall and progression-free survival time. Integration of cognitive neuroscience and neuropsychological evaluations at critical points in the care of patients with brain tumors guides physicians and allied health personnel regarding the multifaceted treatment options that are important at specific points during the disease [5, 19, 21].

Preoperative assessments of NCF may be integrated with neurosurgical procedures used to predict and minimize cognitive morbidity from surgery (e.g., neurocognitive tests, functional MRI, and intraoperative mapping). The early identification of issues that might interfere with cognitive and neuroscience tests, such as inadequate attention, aphasia, or anxiety, as well as specific neurocognitive patterns critical for the interpretation of functional MRI and intraoperative mapping (e.g., nondominant hemisphere language representation) can optimize functional outcome. Perhaps most importantly, NCF performance preoperatively can be used to predict risk of cognitive decline as a function of surgery. For example, in patients with gliomas involving the left temporal lobe, an absence of deficits in the domains of language and verbal memory at presurgical baseline evaluation suggests that the individual may be at increased risk of suffering a surgically induced deficit in those functions. In contrast, patients who have deficits preoperatively tend to show less change as a function of surgery. Many patients who present with brain tumors move quickly to surgical intervention and are experiencing numerous fluctuating factors that affect NCF (e.g., seizures or postictal cognitive changes, a new treatment with steroids or anti-epileptic drugs, and the stress of hospitalization and newly discovered brain mass). Thus, preoperative cognitive assessments are ideally brief and focused on very specific questions [5].

Postoperative NCF evaluation can be used to characterize subacute deficits that may benefit from treatment. The timing of postoperative assessments depends on patient needs and may occur immediately after surgery if the planning of inpatient rehabilitation is necessary. More commonly, a certain amount of time for postsurgical recovery is appropriate, and a comprehensive neuropsychologic evaluation can be conducted on an outpatient basis as the patient receives diagnostic information and makes decisions concerning adjuvant treatment. Postoperative evaluations at this point may be helpful to identify specific cognitive issues that can become targets of outpatient treatment and may play an important role in identifying needs regarding return to work or support in high-level activities of daily living, such as medication management, financial decision-making, and driving [5].

Long-term monitoring of NCF with serial evaluations at regular intervals is helpful as a part of comprehensive brain tumor management. Cognitive impairments can have a more significant impact on quality of life than other neurologic symptoms, and one of the goals of ongoing monitoring is to mitigate the negative impacts of NCF on quality of life. Survivors of brain tumors are at risk for NCF decline caused by tumor recurrence and progression, effects of treatment (chemotherapy and radiation therapy), and neurologic or medical complications of their illness (seizures and cerebrovascular insults). Patients with a history of radiation therapy to the brain are at particular risk for NCF decline due to progressive leukoencephalopathy, often arising months or years after treatment, which requires an increased level of management to provide support for patients and caregivers. Not only do longitudinal evaluations provide practical input for management, but the inclusion of periodic NCF assessments is also a method of monitoring for disease progression or the emergence of post-treatment complications [10, 22, 23].

6 Management of Neurocognitive Symptoms

Unfortunately, there are no specific guidelines for management of NCF symptoms in patients with brain tumors. Although the National Comprehensive Cancer Network (NCCN) has provided guidelines for the management of cognitive symptoms as part of cancer survivorship, these apply explicitly to non–central nervous system cancers and treatments [20]. Efforts are underway to update NCCN central nervous system guidelines to support appropriate follow-up of the neurocognitive aspects of glioma and other central nervous system tumor/treatment-related complications. Specific options to improve NCF outcomes in patients with brain tumors may include preventative measures, rehabilitative efforts, and pharmacologic interventions [5].

6.1 The Role of Neuroscience and Neuropsychological Feedback with Recommendations

The transition point between assessment and management of neurocognitive symptoms occurs during the cognitive neuropsychological evaluation feedback sessions. The feedback session is a therapeutic intervention that gives the patient and family a greater understanding and sense of control over their symptoms, thereby reducing anxiety. Feedback sessions include individualized recommendations based on the patient's pattern of cognitive strength and weakness. Specific cognitive strategies and environmental modifications are recommended, which may allow a patient to independently address the NCF issues arising in their daily activities. These recommendations can also be used to develop accommodations at work or school that may enable an individual to achieve success in those pursuits despite NCF deficits. In cases where NCF deficits are the cause of disability, an unfortunate but not uncommon occurrence for patients with brain tumors, the objective quantification provided by neuropsychological evaluations may be critical to demonstrate deficits and allow access to benefits. Non-neurologic factors contributing to NCF impairment may also be targeted in the recommendations of a neuropsychological evaluation. When symptoms of depression or anxiety are identified as part of the standardized assessment of mood and emotional functioning, the neuropsychologist may refer the patient to mental health services. When issues of sleep disturbance arise, education in the use of sleep hygiene strategies or referral for a formal sleep evaluation may be offered [5, 24, 25].

6.2 Prevention

Proactive efforts to prevent neurologic injury from treatment and increased focus on mitigating neurotoxicity of cancer therapy have led to considerable improvements in NCF outcomes in recent years. These efforts were built upon early work by Meyers et al. (2000), who demonstrated the feasibility and importance of integrating NCF outcomes in clinical trials [17]. As noted earlier, preoperative NCF assessment is often integrated with functional MRI, diffusion tensor imaging to identify critical fiber tracts, intraoperative mapping to assist with planning, and reducing the risk of cognitive morbidity from surgery [17].

In recent years, multiple strategies have been integrated into brain radiation therapy to reduce the risk of NCF sequelae. It has been demonstrated convincingly that the use of focal radiation therapy through stereotactic radiosurgery leads to better NCF outcomes than whole-brain radiation therapy without compromising overall or progression-free survival. As a result, use of focal radiation therapy for solitary or multiple brain metastases is considered the standard of care at this time for patients with limited metastatic disease in the brain [26]. When whole-brain radiation therapy is necessary, the use of hippocampal-sparing treatment, in which the field is tailored to avoid the hippocampal region—critical for memory and neuroplasticity—has been shown to reduce NCF morbidity [27]. Similarly, the use of neuroprotectant strategies when delivering radiation therapy is frequently recommended. Administration of *N*-methyl-D-aspartate receptor antagonist memantine improved cognitive outcomes in patients undergoing whole-brain radiation therapy, and subsequent studies have found that this treatment can be combined with hippocampal-sparing whole-brain radiation therapy to further reduce the risk of NCF decline [5, 26, 27].

6.3 Rehabilitation

Cognitive rehabilitation is a therapy modality that includes explicit instruction in cognitive compensatory strategies, the use of assistive devices to support daily functioning, and in some instances, cognitive exercise to promote brain recovery and maintain brain health. Studies of cognitive rehabilitation in patients with brain tumors have generally demonstrated a positive impact on NCF performance as well as good satisfaction on the part of patients and their families

[28]. Most of these trials have been small and lacked control groups, leading to some limitations in the strength of the literature. Nonetheless, methods that use individualized therapy based on the use of compensatory strategies and supportive devices have resulted in small to moderate improvements in the targeted cognitive functions based on objective testing and/or subjective report. Other studies have used computerized methods to deliver cognitive strategy training or to provide cognitive stimulation and have shown some benefits in terms of attention and processing speed on cognitive tests, though the degree to which these benefits transfer to real-life activities is unknown [27–29].

Physical exercise–based interventions have shown consistent benefits in survivors of pediatric brain tumors, and more recent studies have begun to demonstrate the potential for benefit in adults as well. For example, a study of physical exercise, as compared with an active control condition, demonstrated slight improvements in some aspects of performance-based and self-reported cognitive function, as well as quality of life benefits [30]. Although this literature is limited, there are other reasons to believe that exercise is an important aspect of overall care for patients with brain tumors. Thus, integrating a safe and tolerable exercise routine is a recommended strategy to optimize brain health in all patients with cancer, including those with brain tumors. In those with physical limitations such as hemiparesis, gait disturbance, or visuospatial dysfunction, engaging a physical or occupational therapist to develop a safe and effective exercise strategy may be necessary [5, 30].

7 Management of Additional Factors Contributing to Neurocognitive Function Symptoms

In addition to direct treatment of NCF using rehabilitation or medication, it is important to recognize that numerous neurologic and non-neurologic factors can contribute to cognitive problems in patients with brain tumors. The most prominent factors include fatigue and mood, both of which have strong inter-relationships with individual experiences of NCF. In patients with considerable fatigue, insomnia, excessive daytime sleepiness, or other sleep disorders, integration of sleep studies and treatment of relevant issues is important to optimize NCF. Similarly, disorders of mood, anxiety, and other psychiatric symptoms are common in patients with brain tumors and correlate highly with subjective NCF symptoms. Thus, careful assessment and treatment of cognitive neuroscience and psychological symptoms is an important part of NCF management, with many effective evidence-based strategies available [5, 31].

7.1 Neurocognitive Testing

Neurocognitive testing is a way to measure brain function non-invasively. It is used to assess important aspects of cognition: attention, memory, language, reaction time, perception, etc. This testing is focused on providing small tasks that directly measure those aspects. The different tests are specifically designed to measure aspects of brain function. Neurocognitive testing provides a standardized way to understand the overall brain health of an individual. The tests are objective, and the scores provide a method to compare a person's functioning to the rest of the population, or against themselves at a previous time [32].

Cognitive neuroscience and neuropsychological assessments are designed to measure cognitive functions in both healthy and clinical populations and remain important tools for research studies, clinical diagnoses, patient outcomes, and intervention monitoring. The current standard for testing an individual's cognitive functioning is through conventional validated pencil-paper neuropsychological tests that are administered one-on-one in a clinic or lab setting by a trained psychometrician or cognitive neuropsychologist [32–34].

Computerized administration of clinical instruments is not an entirely new phenomenon and the application of computers to the evaluation of cognition has been studied previously with advances in technology, computerized neuropsychological tests (cNPTs) have been able to address several shortcomings of conventional testing methods. Key advantages of cNPTs over pencil-paper assessments include: (1) consistency in administration and scoring, (2) ability to generate numerous alternate forms for repeated testing, (3) precise stimulus control, (4) ability to record multiple components of a participant's response, (5) adaptability of difficulty levels, (6) decreased cost of administration, (7) increased access for a broader population which can lead to greater diversity among subjects, patients, and normative databases, and (8) ability to run larger validation and reliability studies leading to larger, more accurate normative databases. In their relatively short history, cNPTs have proven advantageous compared to pencil-paper neuropsychological tests, lowering the cost of testing, and expanding their utility and potential applications [32, 35, 36].

At a minimum, cNPTs should provide a set of tests with a range of assessment capabilities that are consistent with a well-defined purpose. In addition, cNPTs must have supporting data to demonstrate response characteristics, reliability, and validity like traditional pencil-paper assessments or other validated cNPTs. Data from published reports have supported the validity, reliability, and feasibility of the use of cNPTs in both clinical and research settings [35, 37].

The NeuroCognitive Performance Test (NCPT; Lumos Labs, Inc.) is a brief, repeatable, web-based platform of cognitive assessments intended to measure functioning across several cognitive domains including working memory, visuospatial memory, psychomotor speed, fluid and logical reasoning, response inhibition, numerical calculation, selective and divided attention [38, 39]. To date, the platform includes 18 subtests that are online adaptations of widely used conventional neuropsychological tests. The NCPT is being developed as an assessment tool applicable to a broad population. In clinical research, the NCPT could have specific utility as a screening tool for entering participants into trials, or as an outcome measure to support efficacy; in clinical settings, it could aid in the diagnosis of cognitive impairment and monitor cognitive change over time [35, 39]. The NCPT platform is modular, and the subtests can be arranged into customized batteries. Eight subtests and several analyses to demonstrate NCPT battery as a measure of cognitive performance are presented below [32].

7.2 Subtests

1. Arithmetic Reasoning is designed to assess numerical problem-solving ability and requires the participant to respond as quickly and accurately as possible to arithmetic problems written in words (e.g., "Four plus two") The primary measure is the number of correct responses minus the number of incorrect responses in 45 seconds [32].
2. Digit Symbol Coding is based on the Digit Symbol Substitution Task and assesses processing speed. The subtest lasts 90 Seconds and participants are required to match a series of numbers that correspond to randomly generated symbols. The primary measure is the number of correct responses minus the number of incorrect responses [34].
3. Forward and Reverse Memory Span assess visual short-term and working memory, respectively, and are based on the Corsi Blocks tasks. These subtests require participants to recall a sequence of randomized spatial locations in either forward or reverse order. The subtest concludes when three consecutive errors on one sequence length are made. The primary measure is the number of correct responses [32].
4. Grammatical Reasoning is based on Baddeley's Grammatical Reasoning Test and is designed to assess cognitive flexibility and reasoning. The subtest lasts 45 s and requires participants to evaluate potentially confusing grammatical statements rapidly and accurately. The primary measure is the number of correct responses minus the number of incorrect responses [35].

5. Progressive Matrices are based on established matrix reasoning assessments and are designed to assess problem-solving and fluid reasoning. The subtest lasts up to 17 trials or concludes when three consecutive errors are made. The primary measure is the number of correct responses [34].
6. Trail Making A and [6] Trail Making B assess attention and processing speed and are based on the Army Individual Test Battery and the Halstead-Reitan Battery (In Trail Making A participants are required to click on a sequential series of encircled numbers from 1 to 24. Task requirements are similar for Trail Making B except the circles include both numbers and letters, and the participant must alternate sequentially between numbers and letters. For both Trail Making A and B, the primary measure is completion time [39].

Based on the cognitive domains captured by the subtests, the factors can be grouped with the following labels: (1) Mental Flexibility [40], Digit Symbol Coding, Arithmetic Reasoning, and Grammatical Reasoning (2) Memory: Forward Memory Span and Reverse Memory Span and (3) Attention and Speed of Processing: Trail Making A and Trail Making B Progressive Matrices, which did not group under these labels, is a measure of fluid intelligence [32].

7.3 The Advantages of Neurocognitive Testing

Neurocognitive testing has several advantages over more invasive tests: There is shorter test time to complete, and unlike very costly brain scans, or surgeries that involve risks, this kind of testing can be done at a desk or on a tablet. Collectively, the scores can be used to measure brain function, and in a clinical setting are often used for the diagnosis of problems, such as concussion, dementia, or learning disabilities. Neurocognitive testing can help detect problems *early on.* Early detection of concussion and dementia are commonly missed but can be prevented because they're accompanied by subtle changes in attention, perception, and hand-eye skills. Neurocognitive testing can uncover the patterns that enable detection and tracking through time, which can establish a baseline of cognition in mild cognitive dementia, or assess recovery after a concussion [41].

Neurocognitive testing has been in use for a long time. Traditionally, it has been done with paper and pencil, however, in recent years computerized neurocognitive tests are even more sensitive and more efficient than traditional tests. We can capture precise reaction times, randomize trials, keep attention focused, be consistent, and score tests objectively. Having the ability to track cognitive health throughout an individual's lifetime enables a deeper understanding of brain health and promotes early action [32, 33].

7.4 Innovation in Neurocognitive Tests

Recently, innovative advanced imaging technologies have been used to address complex brain issues. The new technologies are highly sensitive and can provide detailed insights about the locations of brain impairments and thus enhances surgical outcomes. During surgery, a neuropsychiatrist performs the tests and evaluates a wide range of linguistic and non-linguistic functions of the patient. Some of the nonlanguage functions include attention, higher-level problem-solving, and multitasking.

8 Conclusion

Monitoring NCF in the care of patients with brain tumors is best accomplished via a combination of cognitive screening tools administered in clinic and routine inquiry regarding cognitive concerns of the patient and, when possible, patient's known contacts. Integration of formal neuropsychological assessments at critical points in patient care and over the long term improves sensitivity to NCF issues and changes. Feedback on this kind of assessment provides an opportunity to develop a treatment plan for

NCF. In addition to preventative measures that have been adopted in neurosurgery and radiation oncology, treatment options include cognitive rehabilitation and pharmacotherapy. Interventions to address additional issues, such as problems with sleep, fatigue, and mood, can also lead to improved NCF. Consistent application of these assessment and treatment modalities can improve quality of life and overall outcome throughout the course of disease for patients with brain tumors.

References

1. Horwitz B, Tagamets MA, McIntosh AR. Neural modeling, functional brain imaging, and cognition. Trends Cogn Sci. 1999;3(3):91–8.
2. Sachdev PS, Blacker D, Blazer DG, Ganguli M, Jeste DV, Paulsen JS, Petersen RC. Classifying neurocognitive disorders: the DSM-5 approach. Nat Rev Neurol. 2014;10(11):634–42. https://doi.org/10.1038/nrneurol.2014.181.
3. Aron AR. The neural basis of inhibition in cognitive control. Neuroscientist. 2007;13(3):214–28. https://doi.org/10.1177/1073858407299288.
4. Chaytor N, Schmitter-Edgecombe M. The ecological validity of neuropsychological tests: a review of the literature on everyday cognitive skills. Neuropsychol Rev. 2003;13(4):181–97. https://doi.org/10.1023/b:nerv.0000009483.91468.fb.
5. Parsons MW, Dietrich J. Assessment and management of cognitive symptoms in patients with brain tumors. Am Soc Clin Oncol. 2021;41:e90–9. https://doi.org/10.1200/EDBK_320813.
6. Bressler SL, Tognoli E. Operational principles of neurocognitive networks. Int J Psychophysiol. 2006;60(2):139–48. https://doi.org/10.1016/j.ijpsycho.2005.12.008.
7. Bressler SL, Kelso JS. Cortical coordination dynamics and cognition. Trends Cogn Sci. 2001;5(1):26–36.
8. Racine CA, Li J, Molinaro AM, Butowski N, Berger MS. Neurocognitive function in newly diagnosed low-grade glioma patients undergoing surgical resection with awake mapping techniques. Neurosurgery. 2015;77(3):371–9. https://doi.org/10.1227/NEU.0000000000000779.
9. Tucha O, Smely C, Preier M, Lange KW. Cognitive deficits before treatment among patients with brain tumors. Neurosurgery. 2000;47(2):324–34. https://doi.org/10.1097/00006123-200008000-00011.
10. Taphoorn MJ, Klein M. Cognitive deficits in adult patients with brain tumours. Lancet Neurol. 2004;3(3):159–68.
11. Talacchi A, d'Avella D, Denaro L, Santini B, Meneghelli P, Savazzi S, Gerosa M. Cognitive outcome as part and parcel of clinical outcome in brain tumor surgery. J Neuro-Oncol. 2012;108(2):327–32.
12. Herbet G, Duffau H. Awake craniotomy and bedside cognitive mapping in neurosurgery. In: Neurosurgical neuropsychology. Cambridge, MA: Academic; 2019. p. 113–38.
13. Bonifazi S, Passamonti C, Vecchioni S, Trignani R, Martorano PP, Durazzi V, et al. Cognitive and linguistic outcomes after awake craniotomy in patients with high-grade gliomas. Clin Neurol Neurosurg. 2020;198:106089.
14. Satoer D, Visch-Brink E, Dirven C, Vincent A. Glioma surgery in eloquent areas: can we preserve cognition? Acta Neurochir. 2016;158(1):35–50. https://doi.org/10.1007/s00701-015-2601-7.
15. Santini B, Talacchi A, Squintani G, Casagrande F, Capasso R, Miceli G. Cognitive outcome after awake surgery for tumors in language areas. J Neuro-Oncol. 2012;108(2):319–26. https://doi.org/10.1007/s11060-012-0817-4.
16. Coomans MB, van der Linden SD, Gehring K, Taphoorn M. Treatment of cognitive deficits in brain tumour patients: current status and future directions. Curr Opin Oncol. 2019;31(6):540–7. https://doi.org/10.1097/CCO.0000000000000581.
17. Meyers CA, Hess KR, Yung WK, Levin VA. Cognitive function as a predictor of survival in patients with recurrent malignant glioma. J Clin Oncol. 2000;18(3):646–50. https://doi.org/10.1200/JCO.2000.18.3.646.
18. Folstein MF, Folstein SE, McHugh PR. "Mini-mental state": a practical method for grading the cognitive state of patients for the clinician. J Psychiatr Res. 1975;12(3):189–98.
19. Meyers CA, Hess KR. Multifaceted end points in brain tumor clinical trials: cognitive deterioration precedes MRI progression. Neuro-Oncology. 2003;5(2):89–95.
20. Stavinoha PL, Askins MA, Powell SK, Pillay Smiley N, Robert RS. Neurocognitive and psychosocial outcomes in pediatric brain tumor survivors. Bioengineering. 2018;5(3):73.
21. Noll KR, Bradshaw ME, Rexer J, Wefel JS. Neuropsychological practice in the oncology setting. Arch Clin Neuropsychol. 2018;33(3):344–53.
22. DeAngelis LM, Delattre JY, Posner JB. Radiation-induced dementia in patients cured of brain metastases. Neurology. 1989;39(6):789.
23. Tallet AV, Azria D, Barlesi F, Spano JP, Carpentier AF, Gonçalves A, Metellus P. Neurocognitive function impairment after whole brain radiotherapy for brain metastases: actual assessment. Radiat Oncol. 2012;7(1):1–8.
24. Gorske TT. Therapeutic neuropsychological assessment: a humanistic model and case example. J Humanist Psychol. 2008;48(3):320–39.
25. Noll KR, Bradshaw ME, Weinberg JS, Wefel JS. Neurocognitive functioning is associated with functional independence in newly diagnosed patients with temporal lobe glioma. Neuro-Oncol Pract. 2018;5(3):184–93.

26. Brown PD, Jaeckle K, Ballman KV, Farace E, Cerhan JH, Anderson SK, et al. Effect of radiosurgery alone vs radiosurgery with whole brain radiation therapy on cognitive function in patients with 1 to 3 brain metastases: a randomized clinical trial. JAMA. 2016;316(4):401–9.
27. Attia A, Page BR, Lesser GJ, Chan M. Treatment of radiation-induced cognitive decline. Curr Treat Options in Oncol. 2014;15(4):539–50.
28. Bergo E, Lombardi G, Pambuku A, Della Puppa A, Bellu L, D'avella D, Zagonel V. Cognitive rehabilitation in patients with gliomas and other brain tumors: State of the art. Biomed Res Int. 2016;2016:3041824.
29. Gehring K, Sitskoorn MM, Gundy CM, Sikkes SA, Klein M, Postma TJ, et al. Cognitive rehabilitation in patients with gliomas: a randomized, controlled trial. J Clin Oncol. 2009;27(22):3712–22.
30. Sahnoune I, Inoue T, Kesler SR, Rodgers SP, Sabek OM, Pedersen SE, et al. Exercise ameliorates neurocognitive impairments in a translational model of pediatric radiotherapy. Neuro-Oncology. 2018;20(5):695–704.
31. Litofsky NS, Resnick AG. The relationships between depression and brain tumors. J Neuro-Oncol. 2009;94(2):153–61.
32. Morrison GE, Simone CM, Ng NF, Hardy JL. Reliability and validity of the NeuroCognitive performance test, a web-based neuropsychological assessment. Front Psychol. 2015;6:1652. https://doi.org/10.3389/fpsyg.2015.01652.
33. Williams LM, Simms E, Clark CR, Paul RH, Rowe D, Gordon E. The test-retest reliability of a standardized neurocognitive and neurophysiological test battery: "neuromarker". Int J Neurosci. 2005;115(12):1605–30.
34. Williams JE, McCord DM. Equivalence of standard and computerized versions of the raven progressive matrices test. Comput Hum Behav. 2006;22(5):791–800.
35. Gur RC, Richard J, Hughett P, Calkins ME, Macy L, Bilker WB, et al. A cognitive neuroscience-based computerized battery for efficient measurement of individual differences: standardization and initial construct validation. J Neurosci Methods. 2010;187(2):254–62.
36. Kane RL, Kay GG. Computerized assessment in neuropsychology: a review of tests and test batteries. Neuropsychol Rev. 1992;3(1):1–117. https://doi.org/10.1007/BF01108787.
37. Goel V. Anatomy of deductive reasoning. Trends Cogn Sci. 2007;11(10):435–41. https://doi.org/10.1016/j.tics.2007.09.003.
38. Richardson JT. Measures of short-term memory: a historical review. Cortex. 2007;43(5):635–50.
39. Keefe RS, Goldberg TE, Harvey PD, Gold JM, Poe MP, Coughenour L. The brief assessment of cognition in schizophrenia: reliability, sensitivity, and comparison with a standard neurocognitive battery. Schizophr Res. 2004;68(2–3):283–97.
40. Richardson D, Matlock T. The integration of figurative language and static depictions: an eye movement study of fictive motion. Cognition. 2007;102(1):129–38.
41. Kiely KM. Cognitive function. In: Michalos AC, editor. Encyclopedia of quality of life and well-being research. Dordrecht: Springer; 2014. https://doi.org/10.1007/978-94-007-0753-5_426.

Correction to: History of Awake Craniotomy <Awake Craniotomy, History>

Hadi Digaleh and Mahshid Fallahpour

Correction to:
Chapter 1 in: A. Pour-Rashidi, J. Aarabi (eds.),
The Principles of Successful Awake Craniotomy,
https://doi.org/10.1007/978-981-99-2985-6_1

The author's name was inadvertently published with errors. In Chapter 1, the correct name is **Hadi Digaleh**, while it was mistakenly written as **Dagaleh**. This error has been corrected.

The updated version of the chapter can be found at:
https://doi.org/10.1007/978-981-99-2985-6_1

A. Pour-Rashidi, J. Aarabi (eds.), *The Principles of Successful Awake Craniotomy*,
https://doi.org/10.1007/978-981-99-2985-6_11

GPSR Compliance

The European Union's (EU) General Product Safety Regulation (GPSR) is a set of rules that requires consumer products to be safe and our obligations to ensure this.

If you have any concerns about our products, you can contact us on ProductSafety@springernature.com

In case Publisher is established outside the EU, the EU authorized representative is:

Springer Nature Customer Service Center GmbH
Europaplatz 3
69115 Heidelberg, Germany

Batch number: 10731385

Printed by Printforce, the Netherlands